Pa

Developing Clinical Skills
in Dysphagia

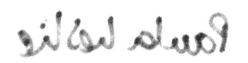

Library of Congress Cataloguing in Publication Data
British Library Cataloguing in Publication Data
A catalogue record for this book is available from the British Library
Cover design: Jim Wilkie
Project management, typesetting and design: J&R Publishing Services Ltd, Guildford,
Surrey, UK; www.jr-publishingservices.co.uk

Printed and bound by CPI Group (UK) Ltd, Croydon, CR0 4YY

Developing Clinical Skills in Dysphagia

A guide for speech and language therapists

Naomi Cocks and Celia Harding
(Editors)

J&R Press Ltd

Contents

Preface

Welcome to *Developing Clinical Skills in Dysphagia*. This guide has been prepared for clinical educators/supervisors in order to help them to support students and newly-qualified therapists who are studying and working in settings where there is a focus on dysphagia. The guide is a supplement to *The Dysphagia Placement Workbook* which has been designed to be used by students and newly-qualified therapists when developing skills in dysphagia. The guide includes the following:

- The rationale for the workbook and how the quoted papers in the accompanying workbook can supplement student learning

- Reports from clinicians about how to use the workbook and how to support students and newly-qualified therapists develop clinical skills

- Suggested ways to support students with clinical documentation

- Templates for case history taking with both paediatric and adult clients

- A DVD with a demonstration of how to prepare for a videofluoroscopic swallowing study, a tour of a videofluoroscopy suite, a demonstration of how to do a videofluoroscopic swallowing study, videofluoroscopic swallowing studies of a normal swallow, an elderly swallow and an impaired swallow, a demonstration of an oral motor assessment and swallow screen, and a demonstration of how to make thickened fluids

- Instructions about how to use the DVD alongside activities in the workbook

- Additional suggested learning activities and projects so that students give something back to your service

- Answers to the Pre-Placement Quizzes from *The Dysphagia Placement Workbook*

The guide and the workbook were developed as part of a research project that ran at City University London in 2009–2010. This arose out of the need expressed by many Clinical Educators (CEs) to develop dysphagia placement opportunities for student speech and language therapists (SSLTs).

Eating, drinking and swallowing disorders within both adult and paediatric populations are identified as being a substantial percentage of a speech and language therapist's caseload (Van der Gaag, McLoone & Reid, 1999). Specific placement and teaching opportunities for students to develop within this area are essential in order for practitioners to be competent providers of health care and to meet the needs of an evolving and complex caseload. The concept, guide and workbook are a step towards addressing this issue.

As part of evolving this concept, it was felt that the current models of student placements could not always provide a suitable learning environment that would help developing practitioners gain any consolidated learning within the field of dysphagia. As part of the research project, a five day 'Dysphagia Intensive Placement' was developed to try and focus on a dysphagia caseload within both acute and community settings, and also paediatric and adult settings.

The supplementary workbook was designed to be used by students whilst on the Dysphagia Intensive Placement. It was developed and refined before and during the research project and was an integral part of the learning experience. The activities in the workbook were specifically created to ensure that students get the most out of their placements as well as beginning to develop basic competencies in dysphagia. The materials that were developed for this project became the basis for *The Dysphagia Placement Workbook*.

As speech and language therapists who work with adults and children, we designed this book and the workbook to be used with a range of populations (both paediatric and adult). It is also suitable for a range of settings (e.g. acute, rehabilitation hospital and community). The guide and workbook are also designed with both UK and Australian students and newly-qualified therapists in mind and therefore refer to relevant policy and guidelines within these countries at the time of print. For ease of expression, the UK term 'speech and language therapist' instead of the Australian term 'speech pathologist' has been used throughout. Similarly, the term 'clinical educator' (or CE) instead of 'supervisor' has been used throughout.

Thanks are extended to particular speech and language therapists who have been involved with this venture and we are very grateful to them for their support. This project would not have been so successful without the help of: Camille Paynter, Nina Bharania, Helen Cockerill, Lizzie Nash, Stacey Lawrence, Annie Aloysius, Lesley Baker, Michelle Miles, Emma Leach and Julie Wright, as well as many other clinicians (there are too many to name but you know who you are) who took part in the research project, gave feedback about the workbook and placement model and who have hosted Dysphagia Intensive Placements for City University London throughout the last few years.

Finally, we hope you enjoy using these materials with speech and language therapy students and newly-qualified therapists within your work environment.

Naomi Cocks and Celia Harding
City University London

References

Van der Gaag, A., McLoone, P., & Reid, D. (1999) Speech and language therapy caseloads in seven districts in the UK. *Journal of Management in Medicine, 13(1)*, 23–32.

1 Using *The Dysphagia Placement Workbook*

Celia Harding and Naomi Cocks

The rationale underpinning *The Dysphagia Placement Workbook* materials

There is an increasing drive to encourage students and clinicians to link theory to practice, and *The Dysphagia Placement Workbook* was developed with this in mind. The workbook includes specific journal references (i.e. peer reviewed evidence in most instances) at the beginning of each activity which helps orientate the student towards research in that particular area. This is followed by questions that link both observation and hands-on experience to the activity and, hence, the research that underpins what the student is evaluating and investigating. The questions are phrased in such a way as to provide opportunities for the student to themselves reflect on the key issues. The activities also help to structure discussion between students/newly-qualified therapists and their clinical educators/supervisors.

It is recognized that, for courses which teach clinical skills alongside academic learning such as speech and language therapy, there is a need for a variety of teaching and learning methods in order to enable students to become able practitioners. Also, there is a need for students to focus on the development of hypothetical thinking skills whilst on placement as a method of tying theory to practice (Lekkas et al., 2007; Lincoln & McAllister, 1993; McAllister, 1997). By introducing the concept of hypothetical thinking alongside both practical and evidence-based resources, the students' early clinical development can be supported in a very structured way. This method is also essential for newly-qualified speech and language therapists as a basis from which they can explore key components of an approach. Such an approach may serve to encourage students and new graduates to develop a working framework to support their own thinking and professional development.

At present, there is no one particular recognizable method or formula that is appropriate for teaching students clinical skills and providing them with the sense that they have learned how to underpin an approach with a rationale

(Horton et al., 2004; Lekkas et al., 2007). Most clinical courses will try a variety of approaches that tap into the range of learning which students undertake, such as deep and surface learning (Scholten, 2001). Recognizing such a difference can provide a variety of teaching methods that support students in their learning experiences with subjects. Traditional didactic methods cannot always ensure that students consolidate and retain new knowledge, and might lead to only surface learning where information is simply memorized or reproduced with little application (Marton & Saljo, 1984; Spencer & Jordan, 1999).

The workbook has attempted to address the issue of supporting students through a range of learning styles. As already indicated, each section is prefaced by a range of relevant peer-reviewed texts that students are encouraged to read before undertaking the activity. Not all papers will need to be read; rather, the reflective approach of identifying the most relevant papers suited to the particular placement is encouraged. Tasks are presented within each section, and there is opportunity for students to discuss with peers and clinical educators (CEs) the relevance of the research that underpins what they have undertaken. Consequently, if much of the intervention rests largely with expert opinion, then this would be a good opportunity for the student or newly-qualified therapist and CE to discuss: (i) how research might be carried out in the identified clinical area; (ii) whether any research in a similar clinical area has been carried out and, if so, whether core components of the method and rationale are relevant to research in the discussed clinical area; (iii) what specifically would be the research question that would need to be asked in order to explore the rationale underpinning a treatment strategy. Students and newly-qualified therapists should also be encouraged to search for more recent research in the particular area. Discussions can then be facilitated in which students and newly-qualified therapists critique the research, explore how the new research findings differ to those of the papers cited, and how the findings might impact on how they work clinically. Thus, the workbook has a format that encourages students to combine a range of approaches to thinking and practical application. Having multi-modal methods of experience can enhance student clinical competence (Horton et al., 2004).

The workbook is set up in such a way so as to create more collaborative learning through joint observation or working with other students (DeClute & Ladyshewsky, 1993). By providing opportunities for students to attend placements with peers, by managing a small caseload and sharing experiences with another student, and by having group discussions with the CEs, they are given more meaningful opportunities to link theory to practice (DeClute &

Ladyshewsky, 1993; Lincoln & McAllister, 1993; McAllister, 2005; Stroshein, Hagler, & May, 2002). This approach enables the notion of team working to become a natural part of clinical management. DeClute and Ladyshewsky (1993) and Baxter and Gray (2001) have carried out research and compared students who were paired on a placement with those who attended a placement on their own. Their findings indicated that the paired placement students had better clinical skill outcomes and competence compared to the students who had attended a solo placement. Better clinical skill outcomes in this study included attributes such as: experience, awareness, knowledge, clinical skills, competence, confidence and interest in the designated clinical area.

The role of the CE cannot be underestimated in the contribution made to student clinical learning. CEs have a vital role in supporting the development of clinical goal-setting skills alongside reflecting about context, input, process and product within a case-based context (Higgs, 1992). The CE is also important as an educator, coach, sponsor, counsellor and confronter, providing students with opportunities to question what they are doing with expert practitioners (Hagler & McFarlane, 1991). CEs need to help students develop clinical skills by engaging with reflective practice (Lincoln & McAllister, 1993; McAllister, 1997). These authors argue that reflective practice is an important method during teaching that enables students to link theory to practice, and also is an important aspect of lifelong learning and professional development.

Therefore, the idea of a placement with a supported workbook is an attempt to integrate a number of specific elements. These include: reflective practice, observation, the evidence underpinning practice, learning from peers and experienced practitioners, and linking theory to practice.

Suggested ways of using the book

The workbook can be used on a number of different levels. It can be used with both students and graduate speech and language therapists who want to develop skills in assessment and management of dysphagia. More prescriptive methods, such as clinical guidelines and competencies provided by professional bodies, give a framework that CEs can use with students and newly-qualified speech and language therapists to guide, monitor and evaluate clinical competence (Stroshein et al., 2002). Using competencies can enable a clear clinical pathway and a planned progression for students and graduate speech and language therapists. This approach will provide a clear and logical method that links component aspects of clinical practice to a more theoretical context (Stroshein et al., 2002).

With the additional resources and the clear use of the evidence base, opportunities for discussion and the prospect of linking theory to practice should be possible. In addition, this should lead to a problem-solving approach based on hypothetical thinking. Such methods have been seen to be effective in research when training students who have a clinical component to their course. Stroshein et al. (2002) wrote about a problem-solving model where students learn analytical skills and strategy management by use of a hypothetical and analytical approach to a clinical case. An interdisciplinary model (Cox et al., 1999) is another method whereby the student takes a client-centred approach to problem solving and developing intervention goals by taking a reflective practice approach. The workbook has been created with these learning issues in mind when working with student and graduate speech and language therapists.

The following two examples illustrate how progression and development can be framed. These examples are supported by quoted evidence from both the Royal College of Speech and Language Therapists (RCSLT) competencies (2003), RCSLT KSF Guidelines (2005) and Speech Pathology Australia (SPA) dysphagia competencies (2004). Details of these can be found at:

Speech Pathology Australia (2004) Dysphagia General: Position Paper (2004). Available on the Speech Pathology Australia webpage: http://www.speechpathologyaustralia.org.au

RCSLT (2003) Reference Framework: Underpinning Competence to Practise: RCSLT Competencies Project: September 2003; London: RCSLT. Available from the Royal College of Speech and Language Therapists webpage: www.rcslt.org/docs/competencies_project

RCSLT (2005) Agenda for Change: Guidance for Speech and Language Therapy staff for developing KSF Outlines. July 2005: London : RCSLT. Available from the Royal College of Speech and Language Therapists webpage: www.rcslt.org/members/publications/VFS_Competencies_KSF_level4v3

EXAMPLE 1

Activity 2: "Mealtime Observation"

Activities begin with a discussion with the clinical educator about current strategies being used with a client prior to observation. Having such a discussion helps a student or newly qualified speech and language therapist to reflect on the age of the client, the client's diagnosis and why such strategies are being used. In addition to this, the student or newly qualified speech and language therapist may wish to explore with the CE any other evidence that supports the approach being used, and make some hypothetical judgements about the case. This can provide an opportunity to discuss the progression of therapy, and key clinical indicators relevant to specific areas.

A clinical example using Activity 2 could be an observation of a neonate in an acute care setting.

A clinical educator may wish to discuss with the student the following features to observe and types of strategies:

- Observation of promoting positive oral experiences through helping the neonate explore their own fingers/nuzzling on a pumped breast/using a pacifier
- Observation of the development of a consistent non-nutritive suck pattern with minimal state changes (i.e. establishing a latch/maintaining a latch/rhythmical sucking bursts/ability to coordinate suck–swallow–breathe cycle
- Observation of how parents and practitioners use non-nutritive sucking during tube feeding
- Observation of an oral trial

The first task in this example is as follows:

> 1. In this activity, you will observe a client during an entire mealtime. Before starting this activity, ask your clinical educator or supervisor for a client that is suitable for this activity. Before observing your client, ask your clinical educator or supervisor if there are any specific management strategies that the client uses as part of their programme, e.g. swallowing manoeuvres, pacing, dummy spoon presentations, slow flow teats, etc. List these below:
>
> Competencies that link to this task are shown in Table 1.

Table 1

RCSLT dysphagia competencies
Family/carer expectations, level of involvement and capacities particularly in the areas of food preparation and nutritional knowledge
Typical sucking......and swallowing patterns in babies
Respiration and impact of dysphagia on respiration
Effects of reflux
Non-oral methods of feeding, e.g. PEG, nasogastric (NG) tube
Effects of oro-aversion/sensory feeding disorders
SPA dysphagia competencies
General observation
Level of alertness/responsiveness
Posture/position
Level of activity/mobility
Presence of nasogastric tube, tracheostomy tube (size, type), gastrostomy tube, intravenous line, central line
Implications of the presence of a nasogastric tube or tracheostomy tube on swallowing function
Ability to be positioned in optimal feeding position and number of staff required to obtain same
Presence of primitive and/or abnormal reflex patterns
Respiratory function at rest and during speech where applicable

2. Describe any equipment that the client is using during their meal, how this equipment helps them with eating or drinking and whether it is effective.

Competencies that link to this task are shown in Table 2.

Table 2

RCSLT dysphagia competencies
Modifying the risk of aspiration
Desensitisation
Compensatory techniques
SPA dysphagia competencies
Impact/use of mealtime equipment

3. Comment on the client's level of independence and whether they can feed themselves or are fed.

Competencies that link to this task are shown in Table 3.

Table 3

RCSLT dysphagia competencies
Influence of environment, positioning, medication, co-existing health concerns, reflux
Feeding method and social issues on infant feeding
SPA dysphagia competencies
Carer participation/skill and knowledge
Knowledge of how feeding dependence vs independence can affect swallowing

4. Comment on the client's posture before the meal.

Competencies that link to this task are shown in Table 4.

Table 4

RCSLT dysphagia competencies
Influence of environment, positioning, medication, co-existing health concerns, reflux

SPA dysphagia competencies
General observation Posture/position

5. Describe the consistency of the food being eaten.

Competencies that link to this task are shown in Table 5.

Table 5

RCSLT dysphagia competencies
Clinically significant signs related to dysphagia status (e.g. overt/silent aspiration) and when to intervene Neonatal observation Maturation of suck–swallow–breathe cycle Oro-motor stimulation

SPA dysphagia competencies
Trial appropriate management strategies (e.g. swallowing manoeuvres – see section on treatment) Impact/use of mealtime equipment

6. Comment on the environment in which the client is eating. Is it noisy? What is the lighting like? Is it in a dining room or are they eating alone?

Competencies that link to this task are shown in Table 6.

Table 6

RCSLT dysphagia competencies
Effects of illness, hospitalization on parental bonding and child development
Developmental care
Foetal development, especially head, neck and face
Neonatal observation
Maturation of suck–swallow–breathe
Oro-motor stimulation
Influence of environment, positioning, medication, co-existing health concerns, reflux
Feeding method and social issues on infant feeding
SPA dysphagia competencies
Carer participation/skill and knowledge

7. Comment on the rate at which the client is fed/feeds themselves and the quantity of the bolus.

Competencies that link to this task are shown in Table 7.

Table 7

RCSLT dysphagia competencies
Influence of environment, positioning, medication, co-existing health concerns, reflux
Feeding method and social issues on infant feeding
Effects of illness, hospitalization on parental bonding and child development
SPA dysphagia competencies
Impact of taste, temperature, size of bolus on swallowing
Impact/use of mealtime equipment
Carer participation/skill and knowledge

8. Comment on whether or not the client becomes tired during the meal. If so, describe what happens.

Competencies that link to this task are shown in Table 8.

Table 8

RCSLT dysphagia competencies
Influence of environment, positioning, medication, co-existing health concerns, reflux
Feeding method and social issues on infant feeding
Effects of illness, hospitalization on parental bonding and child development

SPA dysphagia competencies
General observation
Level of alertness/responsiveness
Level of activity/mobility
Carer participation/skill and knowledge

9. Comment on any features occurring that you feel are indicative of risk. You must inform your clinical educator or supervisor of these risks.

Competencies that link to this task are shown in Table 9.

Table 9

RCSLT dysphagia competencies
Modifying the risk of aspiration
Clinically significant signs related to change in dysphagia status (e.g. overt/silent aspiration) and when to intervene

SPA dysphagia competencies
Education of client, carer or medical team to reduce risk of aspiration and/or improve swallow function
Evaluate risk of aspiration and airway obstruction

10. Does any communication take place during the meal? For example, between the person feeding the client and the client. Describe the communication that occurs. Remember to also include any non-verbal communication.

Competencies that link to this task are shown in Table 10.

Table 10

RCSLT dysphagia competencies
Influence of environment, positioning, medication, co-existing health concerns, reflux
Feeding method and social issues on infant feeding
Effects of illness, hospitalization on parental bonding and child development
Social context of mealtimes
SPA dysphagia competencies
Communication status
Carer participation/skill and knowledge

11. Comment on whether the specific management strategies that you listed at the start of this activity were followed. If any were not followed, indicate below why you think they were not followed. You must inform your clinical educator or supervisor if any were not followed.

Competencies that link to this task are shown in Table 11.

Table 11

RCSLT dysphagia competencies
Seeking information and assessing its relevance
Integration of data from different sources
Analysis
Synthesis
Generating hypotheses
Generating viable options
Decision-making
Critical reflection
Evaluation
Reframing issues/calibrating responses according to feedback

SPA dysphagia competencies
Education of client, carer or medical team to reduce risk of aspiration and/or improve swallow function
Evaluate risk of aspiration and airway obstruction
Trial appropriate management strategies

12. If you had the opportunity to observe a client who is dependent for feeding, then try to observe the client being fed by one or more different carers/support workers. Were there any differences? If so, what were the differences?

Competencies that link to this task are shown in Table 12.

Table 12

RCSLT dysphagia competencies
Client context
• Family/carer expectations, level of involvement and capacities, particularly in the areas of food preparation and nutritional knowledge
• Carer networks
• Cultural and religious background
• Quality of life/ethical considerations
Neonatal feeding
• Influence of environment, positioning, medication, co-existing health concerns, reflux, feeding method and social issues on infant feeding

SPA dysphagia competencies
Carer participation/skill and knowledge
The managing speech pathologist should ensure that where training is required for the client or carer to implement a management plan that they are provided with an optimal method to maximize understanding of what is required. This may include use of interpreters, visual and written aids
Integration of significant features gained from background, observations, communication status, clinical assessment, suitability for oral trials, instrumental assessment and swallowing trials

13. From your reading, what are some of the barriers to caregivers' compliance with eating and drinking recommendations?

See Table 12.

14. Are there other professionals who are or need to be involved in this case? If yes, who are they and why should they be involved?

Students and NQTs would be expected to reflect on their teams and discuss the roles of the other practitioners. From RCSLT CQ 3 (2006), students and NQTs could be referred to pages 324 and 328. From Speech Pathology Australia (2004), Dysphagia General: Position Paper section 7 (page 6) on Team Work would be useful as a basis for discussion.

Table 13

RCSLT dysphagia competencies Related to clinical management • Working within a multidisciplinary team
SPA dysphagia competencies Collaboration with multidisciplinary team in provision of recommendations to address nutritional needs, seating and positioning, equipment for meals/feeding, and respiratory health

EXAMPLE 2

Activity 8: Videofluoroscopic Swallowing Study (VFSS)

A clinical example could be an adult, aged 77 years who has dysphagia as a consequence of having a stroke.

As with all the activities in *The Dysphagia Placement Workbook*, the journal articles listed at the beginning of this activity provide evidence that can be added to discussion with a CE prior to observation as well as prior to and after using the video resources. Potential discussion points might involve:

- When is a videofluoroscopic swallowing study not appropriate?

- Radiation risk

- Radiation protection

- Viscosity issues

- Rater-reliability and interpretation

- Relating findings to bedside and/or mealtime assessment

- The challenge of sharing the news with regards to the outcome of a videofluoroscopic swallowing study

- Parents and/or clients who choose not to agree with the outcome of a videofluoroscopic swallowing study

The first task in this example is as follows:

1. Watch a videofluoroscopic swallowing study (VFSS). (a) Were there any signs of dysphagia? If so, what were they?

Competencies that link to this task are shown in Table 14.

Table 14

RCSLT dysphagia competencies/KSF guidelines
Able to identify the following structures at rest in lateral and A/P views: hyoid/pharynx/posterior pharyngeal wall/piriform sinuses/larynx (thyroid/cricoid/arytenoid cartilages); trachea/upper oesophageal sphincter/cervical oesophagus/cervical spine
Demonstrates knowledge of rationale, indications and limitations for performing videofluoroscopic assessment of swallowing

SPA dysphagia competencies
Knowledge of the application and limitations of, and suitability for, videofluoroscopic evaluation
Integration of significant features gained from background, observations, communication status, clinical assessment, suitability for oral trials, instrumental assessment and swallowing trials
Evaluate risk of aspiration and airway obstruction

(b) Comment on the advantages and the disadvantages of the VFSS.

Competencies that link to this task are shown in Table 15.

Table 15

RCSLT dysphagia competencies/KSF guidelines
Demonstrates knowledge of rationale, indications and limitations for performing videofluoroscopic assessment of swallowing
Able to describe rationale for performing an instrumental assessment of swallowing
Able to describe a rationale for performing a videofluoroscopic assessment of swallowing
Able to describe the contra-indications of performing a videofluoroscopic assessment of swallowing
Able to describe the limitations of performing a videofluoroscopic assessment of swallowing

SPA dysphagia competencies

Knowledge of the application and limitations of, and suitability for, videofluoroscopic evaluation

Knowledge of the application, limitations and suitability of the following assessments:

    Fibrotic endoscopic evaluation of swallowing (FEES)

    Cervical auscultation (CA)

    Pharyngeal manometry

    Pulse oximetry

    Ultrasound

    Nuclear scintigraphy

    Blue dye test (Trache clients only)

    Electromyography

(c) If you have access to the results of the client's bedside assessment, then comment on how the VFSS findings compare to the outcomes of the bedside assessment. Do the VFSS findings contribute anything new? If yes, describe them below.

Competencies that link to this task are shown in Table 16.

Table 16

RCSLT dysphagia competencies/KSF guidelines

Demonstrates knowledge of rationale, indications and limitations for performing videofluoroscopic assessment of swallowing

SPA dysphagia competencies

Knowledge of the application and limitations of, and suitability for, videofluoroscopic evaluation

Integration of significant features gained from background, observations, communication status, clinical assessment, suitability for oral trials, instrumental assessment and swallowing trials

Evaluate risk of aspiration and airway obstruction

2. With a peer, script how you would break 'bad news', e.g. the VFSS examination indicates that the client should not eat/feed orally.

Competencies that link to this task are shown in Table 17.

Table 17

RCSLT dysphagia competencies/KSF guidelines
Ability to interpret and report the outcome of the evaluation following the examination with the use of recorded materials
SPA dysphagia competencies
Education of client, carer or medical team to reduce risk of aspiration and/or improve swallow function

Summary

These two examples clearly illustrate the scope of the workbook tasks. Each specific question within the activity can be matched to relevant competencies. Where newly qualified speech and language therapists and students are working towards achieving competencies this could be a method of recording progress.

A comment on references used to support the text

The references at the beginning of each section of the workbook have been carefully selected with the topic in mind and with a focus on clinical practice. It is anticipated that students will not be required to read all of the references in each instance and that some selective assessment will need to take place as to which papers would be beneficial. This in itself is an important learning exercise: learning to prioritize reading that is relevant, and identifying core texts that will support clinical thinking. As already indicated, students may also be encouraged to carry out literature searches to determine whether any new research has been carried out and then this literature search can be used as the basis for further discussion.

To illustrate how the articles may be used to facilitate discussion, we will use **Activity 7, Management**, as an example. The following list includes the references recommended for that chapter:

- Foley, N., Teasell, R., Salter, K., Kruger, E. & Martino, R. (2008) Dysphagia treatment post stroke: A systemic review of randomised controlled trials. *Age and Ageing, 37,* 258–264.

- Harding, C. (2009) An evaluation of the benefits of non-nutritive sucking for premature infants as described in the literature. *Archives of Disease in Childhood, 94(8),* 636–640.

- Hewetson, R. & Singh, S. (2009) The lived experience of mothers of children with chronic feeding and/or swallowing difficulties. *Dysphagia, 24,* 322–332.

- Husseyin, A., Calis, A. & Turgut, S. (2003) A randomized control trial of early oral feeding in laryngectomised patients. *Laryngoscope, 113 (6),* 1076–1079.

- Perry, A., Shaw, M. & Cotton, S. (2003) An evaluation of functional outcomes (speech, swallowing) in patients attending speech pathology after head and neck cancer treatments: Results and analysis at 12 months post intervention. *Journal of Laryngology and Otology, 117(5),* 368–381.

- Pinnington, L. & Hegarty, J. (2000) Effects of consistent food presentation on oral-motor skill acquisition in children with severe neurological impairment. *Dysphagia, 15,* 213–223.

- Robbins, J., Gensler, G., Hind, J., Logemann, J., Lindbald, A., Brandt, D. et al. (2008) Comparison of 2 interventions for liquid aspiration on pneumonia incidence. *Annals of Internal Medicine, 148,* 509–518.

- Robbins, J., Butler, S.G., Daniels, S.K., Gross, R.D., Langmore, S., Lazarus, C.L. et al. (2008) Swallowing and dysphagia rehabilitation: Translating principles of neural plasticity into clinically oriented evidence. *Journal of Speech, Language, and Hearing Research, 51,* S276–S300.

- Schwartz, S., Corredor, J., Fisher-Medina, J., Cohen, J. & Rabinowitz, S. (2001) Diagnosis and treatment of feeding disorders in children with developmental disabilities. *Pediatrics, 108(3),* 671–676.

These references have been selected for their clinical relevance and clinical application, and represent a range across both paediatric and adult caseloads. The **Activity 7: Management** papers cover a range of issues that are essential for a therapist to consider: carer involvement and carer perceptions of intervention (e.g. Hewetson & Singh, 2009); role definition with treatment and dysphagia (e.g. Schwartz et al., 2001); actual interventions that are carried out by speech and language therapists (Foley et al., 2008; Harding, 2009; Husseyin et al., 2003; Perry et al., 2003; Robbins et al., 2008;) and theoretical ideas that underpin interventions (Robbins et al., 2008; Harding, 2009).

Students and newly qualified therapists (NQTs) are expected to be selective about which papers they would wish to read in relation to their placement. It could be pertinent in some instances to reflect on core similarities as well as differences across the age span with management. Such discussions could be a method of helping students and NQTs to formulate views on the current evidence base and the challenges for researchers within a therapeutic context. However, there are some questions and suggested discussion topics which could be core to all of the papers, and could provide additional discussion activities during reflective practice scenarios:

1. Are there key research design aspects of a selection of papers that could be applied to a clinical context, or that could be difficult to evaluate in a clinical setting? What question would you wish to ask and how would you design this research?

2. Are the papers evaluating strategies that speech and language therapists currently use, or are they focusing on strategies that are more challenging to implement in a clinical setting? If you feel that the strategies do not quite represent practice in the workplace, why is this, and how could you go about designing a study that appears to represent practice across the spectrum more accurately?

3. If the papers discussed address one aspect of the caseload being experienced, are there other strategies that relate to the intervention? If so, how would this be evaluated?

4. Do the papers themselves use peer reviewed journals consistently to support their arguments?

5. What are the challenges of the research discussed in relation to engaging with carers, or the clients themselves?

6. What is the range of statistical testing across the papers used? For example, the paper by Hewetson and Singh (2009), which employs phenomenological analysis, could be compared with another paper from the list that uses different analytical methods.

7. Reflect on research that has evaluated aspects of oral motor function in normal populations. An example could be the paper by Potter et al. (2009) that covers a normal population of 150 children and explores tongue strength development. Do normal data bases have useful information for clinicians? What are these benefits? Are there any challenges? What do you know about muscle composition of both the oral tract and the rest of the human body? Why is this knowledge applicable to our understanding of treatment interventions? Are there other papers that look at specific oral-motor aspects relevant to eating and drinking within a normal population? If there are, what are the clinical benefits, if any?

8. The paper by Kleim and Jones (2008) could be recommended for students and NQTs to reflect on treatment in dysphagia. Using the headings or classifications highlighted in this paper, students and NQTs may wish to categorize where they see research fits in relation to their clinical area. There could be opportunities to think about aspects of rationales that underpin therapy, such as congenital versus acquired difficulties, the origin of swallow function in the brain and whether management tries to accommodate the notions of neurology and plasticity.

9. Students and NQTs should also be encouraged to critique the papers' methodology and discuss their limitations. It may also be useful to determine the level of evidence for each intervention study using criteria derived from The Joanna Briggs Institute for Evidence Based Nursing and Midwifery Levels of Evidence (see http://www.joannabriggs.edu. au/Appraise%20Evidence).

References

Baxter, S. & Gray, C. (2001) The application of student-centred learning approaches to clinical education. *International Journal of Language and Communication Disorders, 36,* 396–400.

Cox, P.D., Beaton, C., Bossers, A., Pepper, J. & Gage, M. (1999) Interdisciplinary pilot project to a rehabilitation setting. *Journal of Allied Health,* 28, 25–29.

DeClute, J. & Ladyshewsky, R.K. (1993) Enhancing clinical competence using a collaborative clinical education model. *Physical Therapy, 73(10),* 683–97.

Foley, N., Teasell, R., Salter, K., Kruger, E. & Martino, R. (2008) Dysphagia treatment post stroke: A systemic review of randomised controlled trials. *Age and Ageing, 37,* 258–264.

Hagler, P. & McFarlane, L. (1991) Achieving maximum student potential: The supervisor as coach. *Canadian Journal of Rehabilitation, 5,* 5–16.

Harding, C. (2009) An evaluation of the benefits of non-nutritive sucking for premature infants as described in the literature. *Archives of Disease in Childhood, 94(8),* 636–640.

Hewetson, R. & Singh, S. (2009) The lived experience of mothers of children with chronic feeding and/or swallowing difficulties. *Dysphagia, 24,* 322–332.

Higgs, J. (1992) Managing clinical education: The educator manager and the self-directed learner. *Physiotherapy, 8,* 822–828.

Horton, S., Byng, S., Bunning, K. & Pring, T. (2004) Teaching and learning speech and language therapy skills: The effectiveness of classroom as clinic in speech and language therapy student education. *International Journal of Communication Disorders,* 39, 365–390.

Husseyin, A., Calis, A. & Turgut, S. (2003) A randomized control trial of early oral feeding in laryngectomised patients. *Laryngoscope, 113 (6),* 1076–1079.

Kleim, J.A. & Jones, T.A. (2008) Principles of experience-dependent neural plasticity: Implications for rehabilitation after brain damage. *Journal of Speech, Language and Hearing Research, 51,* S225-S239.

Lekkas, P., Larsen, T., Kumar, S., Grimmer, K., Nyland, L., Chipchase, L., Jull G., Buttrum, P., Carr, L. & Finch, J. (2007) No model of clinical education for physiotherapy students is superior to another: A systematic review. *Australian Journal of Physiotherapy, 53,* 19–28.

Lincoln, M. & McAllister, L. (1993) Facilitating peer learning in clinical education. *Medical Teacher, 15,* 17–25.

Marton, F. & Saljo, R. (1984) Approaches to learning. In F. Marton, D. Hounsell & N. Entwhistle (Eds) *The Experiences of Learning,* Edinburgh: Scottish Academic Press.

McAllister, L. (1997) *Facilitating Learning in Clinical Settings,* Cheltenham: Stanley Thornes.

McAllister, L. (2005) Issues and innovations in clinical education. *International Journal of Speech-Language Pathology, 7(3),* 138–148.

Perry, A., Shaw, M. & Cotton, S. (2003) An evaluation of functional outcomes (speech, swallowing) in patients attending speech pathology after head and neck cancer treatments: Results and analysis at 12 months post intervention. *Journal of Laryngology and Otology, 117(5)*, 368–381.

Pinnington, L. & Hegarty, J. (2000) Effects of consistent food presentation on oral-motor skill acquisition in children with severe neurological impairment. *Dysphagia, 15,* 213–223.

Potter N.L. & Short, R. (2009) Maximal tongue strength in typically developing children and adolescents. *Dysphagia, 24,* 391–397.

Robbins, J., Butler, S.G., Daniels, S.K., Gross, R.D., Langmore, S., Lazarus, C.L. et al. (2008) Swallowing and dysphagia rehabilitation: Translating principles of neural plasticity into clinically oriented evidence. *Journal of Speech, Language, and Hearing Research, 51,* S276–S300, February 2008. doi:10.1044/1092-4388(2008/021).

Robbins, J., Gensler, G., Hind, J., Logemann, J., Lindbald, A., Brandt, D. et al. (2008) Comparison of 2 interventions for liquid aspiration on pneumonia incidence. *Annals of Internal Medicine, 148,* 509–518.

Sholten, I. (2001) Teachers' conceptions of their role in improving students' preparation for clinical work in dysphagia. *American Journal of Speech-Language Pathology, 10,* 343–357.

Spencer, J. & Jordan, R. (1999) Learner centred approaches in medical education. *British Medical Journal, 318,* 1280–1283.

Strohscein, J., Hagler, P. & May, L. (2002) Assessing the need for change in clinical education practices. *Physical Therapy, 82(2),* 160–72.

2 Clinicians' Accounts of Hosting a Dysphagia Placement and Using *The Dysphagia Placement Workbook*

Camille Paynter, Lizzie Nash, Michelle Miles, Helen Cockerill and Nina Bharania

In this chapter, clinicians from a range of settings share their experience of running dysphagia placements and using *The Dysphagia Placement Workbook*. The clinicians share the advantages, the challenges and essential tips for running a dysphagia placement.

An acute hospital environment with adult clients

Camille Paynter

Running a dysphagia placement

When I was approached by City University London to pilot an intensive dysphagia placement, I was immediately interested. I knew there was a need for students to have more opportunities to develop their clinical skills and knowledge in this area. I have personal experience of this type of placement both as a student and a clinical supervisor in Australia and I knew how successful it could be (although in the past I had only one student to supervise, not six!). I was keen to discover whether this style of placement would suit students in the UK and I also saw this as an opportunity to develop my student supervision skills.

My colleagues and manager were supportive of the idea. The acute trust that I was working for at the time have a strong commitment to student education so were also supportive of my request to pilot the project.

Working with six students over five consecutive days was manageable but required advanced planning, a supportive team and the workbook Celia and Naomi from City University London had developed (*The Dysphagia Placement Workbook*). As a department, we decided that I would not carry a full caseload that week and I would be responsible for providing the teaching/tutorial sessions.

I structured the week by devising a clear timetable of daily tasks structured around the department's weekly routine plus the workbook activities, including required resources, and even listed homework tasks! The daily learning outcomes were clearly stated which helped the clinicians plan and students prepare (that way, none of us had any excuse for not being organized). Students attended placement from 9–5 but were usually given independent or group learning tasks from the workbook to complete at the beginning and the end of each day, freeing up clinicians' time for the usual administrative tasks, preparation and feedback meetings.

Students worked in pairs and were supervised by different clinicians each day. We decided in advance to mix both student pairings and clinicians throughout the week. That way, students would benefit from seeing different clinicians work, have the opportunity to learn from a variety of peers and it would prevent any 'cliquey' groups from forming.

Students were given feedback immediately following their sessions. Clinicians met daily (for less than 30 minutes) to discuss each student and de-brief. This also provided an opportunity for the clinicians with less student supervision experience to receive supervision or advice. Final placement feedback was shared between clinicians in order to reduce the workload on one clinician. The daily meetings meant we were familiar with how all the students had progressed, so dividing this task was straightforward.

Using *The Dysphagia Placement Workbook*

The workbook was a fantastic resource. It promoted consistency of experiences for the students (both during paired and individual tasks) and an overall structure to the placement. It also meant there were activities the students could be doing that I didn't have to pre-plan.

The pre-placement activities provided clear foundation tasks for the students. This was helpful to ensure that students commenced the placement with similar knowledge. How they approached and completed these tasks provided us with some initial insights into their strengths and needs. It also made students aware from the outset that the placement involved independent learning and it was their responsibility to be prepared.

I found the workbook very flexible. The activities didn't all have to be completed consecutively and could be timetabled around existing department routine.

We used the observation activities as an opportunity for students to improve their knowledge of what's normal in the aged population. Therefore, these activities were done twice: once to observe older people without dysphagia, and then again observing patients with dysphagia. Not only did this assist their foundation knowledge when doing their clinical assessments but it helped to improve their confidence when interacting with patients for the first time.

Naomi and Celia have since developed and expanded the workbook into a brilliant reference book with up-to-date research and evidence base and many resources. I find it a great asset and really useful for all my students now.

Challenges

Space!

Most departments are pushed to find one or two spare desks for students – but six? We managed by booking meeting rooms for specific teaching sessions and using space in the library or the cafeteria for students to complete workbook tasks.

Caseload management

The intensity of having six students for the whole week did have an impact on how we managed our caseload. However, we had pre-planned that the lead therapist would carry a minimal caseload for the week. This ensured there was a dedicated clinician to manage any student issues and that all patients were seen appropriately.

Making sure patients with communication impairments don't miss out

Having students on a placement specifically focused on dysphagia did mean that patients with communication impairments were at risk of not being seen as often. We tried to manage this in advance by setting up patients with independent therapy programmes or recruiting therapy assistants to help.

Lack of appropriate patients

We certainly hadn't anticipated a lack of appropriate patients. You guessed it – during the whole week only one patient who had had a stroke was admitted. It taught me that you can never plan for everything and that speech and language therapists are flexible and good problem solvers!

Therapy versus intervention

At the end of the placement, all students fed back that they hadn't observed any therapy. This was partly due to the fact that many of the patients seen weren't appropriate for impairment-based therapy. It may also indicate we focused on clinical assessment skills rather than treatment skills. But on reflection, I also realized that my explanations needed to explicitly stress that often the recommendations (that is, diet, bolus or behaviour modification) *are* the interventions. It made me realize that it is important for clinical educators to help students broaden their understanding of what 'therapy' is.

Finding time to give feedback on the workbook tasks

The clinicians found it very challenging to find time in the day to provide feedback on the workbook tasks. We therefore asked the students to conduct this as a group activity and provide peer support which they were able to do at the beginning or end of the day during non-clinician time.

Tips for other clinicians

Feedback: The duplicate book

Finding time for feedback is often challenging. Have you ever felt you'd had plenty of discussion time with a student but at the end of the placement they've said they would have liked more feedback? I have, and that's when I started using the duplicate book. In my experience, when students receive written feedback, not only do they remember it, they also feel the feedback is more substantial.

We used A5 size duplicate books so both student and clinician had a written record of the discussion and learning points. During this placement, students were given feedback immediately following their session. Because students were being supervised by different clinicians throughout the week, this written record was invaluable for handing over information and reviewing their progress.

All of the students on this placement reported they received *frequent* and *sufficient* feedback on their clinical skills, an outcome of which I was particularly proud.

Other Allied Health Professional input

Even though the timetable was tight and there was a lot of speech and language therapy clinical knowledge to cover, we felt it was important for the students to have a basic understanding of the roles of other professionals in managing dysphagia in the acute setting. Our dietetic and physiotherapy colleagues conducted tutorials which the students reported as being valuable experiences.

Exploit the unexpected opportunities

When a patient's family member disagreed with my recommendations, it was a wonderful opportunity to explore complex issues. We had the opportunity to discuss capacity and the Mental Capacity Act (2005), explore ethical issues, quality of life and patient best interest. And as Nina describes in her reflections on running a dysphagia placement in an Adults with Learning Disability community setting, it helped the students to appreciate real life risk management. So don't be afraid of disagreement, it can lead to the most interesting session of the week!

Benefits

There were numerous benefits from running this placement, and I would encourage you to give it a try even if you're unsure. Of course, you don't have to start with six students, but in my experience having a pair of students on a placement like this is probably more manageable than having a single student.

The students on the pilot placement reported they benefited from having a focused learning area for the whole week. Plus, they had the opportunity to apply theory to practice immediately. Not only did they learn from a variety of clinicians but they also had many opportunities for peer learning when working in pairs or during whole group activities. They were exposed to working in the acute hospital environment and to the roles and responsibilities of different professionals. They obtained a basic working knowledge of the structure of healthcare.

This placement is structured, focused on one particular teaching area and has a supportive workbook. Therefore it is an excellent opportunity for clinicians who are inexperienced in student supervision to develop their skills in teaching and supervising in a structured and supported way.

At the end of the placement, every clinician involved reported improved clinical skills and theoretical knowledge in dysphagia.

Some of the benefits to the speech and language therapy department and the clinicians involved in the placement weren't anticipated. One such benefit was team building. Also, my two colleagues reported an increase in confidence in having to carry a senior therapist's caseload when I was completing induction or teaching.

Being involved in the successful piloting of the Intensive Dysphagia Placement for City University London was an excellent experience both professionally and personally. I hope you enjoy your experience.

An acute paediatric hospital setting
Lizzie Nash, Michelle Miles, Helen Cockerill

Scene setting

As a department, we recognize the increased need for students to gain experience in paediatric dysphagia. This area of clinical practice is now an integral part of pre-registration speech and language therapy training. Students frequently request the opportunity to have a paediatric dysphagia placement. Within the department, staff members have been involved in teaching dysphagia to pre-registration students and we wanted to be active participants in developing paediatric dysphagia placements for students.

In the UK, the role of the speech and language therapist in acute paediatric settings has become more established. There has been a shift from a patchy service provided by community therapists visiting hospital wards to therapists becoming established and integral team members within an acute setting, at least within the large teaching hospitals. Having therapists as part of a multidisciplinary team can have a positive impact on reducing hospital stay and re-admission.

Traditionally, it hasn't been popular to take students on dysphagia placements, because weekly therapy sessions do not allow a student to gain a sense of continuity of care on a daily basis (e.g. the challenge of orchestrating the weekly therapy sessions with the same patient) or allow an appreciation of the wider multidisciplinary team within acute care. Historically, it has been preferable for clinicians to take students who had established skills in previous placements (i.e. already had established a level of professional experience). Clinicians have previously relied on generic handbooks from academic departments which required adapting to the acute setting and dysphagia. It has been left to the clinician to allocate tasks for the student, which involved careful consideration to the degree of risk/adverse consequence if something went wrong. This has been a drain on clinicians' time and perhaps would mean that students were left to observe rather than access experiential learning opportunities.

Advantages of *The Dysphagia Placement Workbook*

The five day dysphagia intensive placement offered to students from City University London was an elective placement, and we were aware that the competition was high. Consequently, the students who were allocated the placement were highly motivated. This motivation was enhanced by the Pre-Placement Activities in the workbook; students were pre-motivated and had a vested interest to learn.

The workbook provided a clear focus and structure for both the placement and the students' own learning in that clinical area. This promoted independent learning and also had resources to support the clinician's caseload and daily work regime. The knowledge quiz in the workbook provided a baseline measure of the students' knowledge/skills. This enabled the clinician to differentiate tasks to each student's level and jointly set learning goals.

The activities provided specific topics relevant for dysphagia management with questions and literature that guided discussions between clinicians and students. The structure was clear in that it allowed clear boundaries between observation and patient contact, i.e. managing risk of harm. Given the topic base of the workbook which focused on key skills rather than specific populations, it was possible to use with a paediatric population and across a whole range of care groups, e.g. neonates, congenital disorders and acquired brain injury. As a team, we felt it was important that the communication aspect was acknowledged as an integral part of management.

Application to an acute paediatric setting: Challenges and benefits

We would recommend that clinicians considering such a placement to think about any additional texts that are specific to their populations. As a team, we did this as we felt it supplemented the literature in the workbook. For example, as we work with infants we discussed and shared literature on breast feeding, early infant assessment of feeding and paediatric tracheostomy care.

Because we are a large team, we found that it helped with overall management to have a named therapist as the clinical educator. On placement, thought needs to be given to orientation of the student to the environment and any relevant policies within the organization, such as safeguarding children, issues of confidentiality, and so on.

It was recognized that we did actually place more emphasis on communication with some children, particularly with those who have behavioural feeding difficulties and those with more complex needs, e.g. early stages of recovery from brain injury. Because the workbook is generic, we felt that we needed to enhance the topic areas by having more emphasis on developmental norms for language development and communication generally, as well as reiterating the development of eating and drinking skills.

Students were required to adjust quickly to the unpredictable nature of the acute paediatric placement. Because of this, it was important to stress to the students that it wasn't always possible to carry out planned activities, and that although the placement was a week, not all of the activities had to be completed before the end of the placement. Challenges such as this enabled clinicians and students to reflect on the adaptable working that clinicians are expected to do in an acute setting.

We were aware that students may only have experienced community placements prior to the Dysphagia Intensive Placement. With this in mind, we felt that emotional preparation and support was important: e.g. preparing the student for environments such as PICU (Paediatric Intensive Care Unit), NICU (Neonatal Intensive Care Unit); allowing students time to reflect on bereavement; breaking bad news; issues with palliative care cases, and so on. Developing awareness of the progression of cases from acute to community settings and the requirements of liaison were important aspects that needed to be stressed within our setting. This gave students the opportunity to reflect on relevant team members' roles as well as on their own professional boundaries. We were also able to discuss specific issues relevant to our setting, such as differences in levels of intervention within acute care compared to community settings.

We valued having access to staff at City University London to discuss queries and for general feedback. As part of the support offered, we were aware that we could contact the placement coordinators if we felt we had any professional standards issues. Generally, we felt the intense nature of the placement gave students insight into caseload management that a weekly placement would never allow. Additionally, given the quick turnover of in-patients and the rapidly changing nature of paediatric conditions on a day-to-day basis, the intensive nature of this programme suited our team.

A community setting for adults with learning disabilities
Nina Bharania

Challenges of running a dysphagia placement in this setting

Initially, I thought the concept of running a placement that focused specifically on dysphagia sounded quite challenging. Some of my first thoughts were: "Will there be enough dysphagia cases for them to observe; will there be appropriate cases that are exciting enough; what will the students do exactly?" My interpretation was that I would need to pack in as many assessments as possible for the students to observe. Knowing that this was not realistic, I soon realized that the best thing was for the students to see what therapists actually did in the context of supporting adults with learning disabilities in the community.

The students gave me the general impression that they viewed adult dysphagia more in terms of acute-based hospital work, i.e. giving patients teaspoons of water, listening to the swallow with a stethoscope and recommending nil by mouth frequently. This is very different from observing whole mealtimes in people's homes (and sometimes in more than one environment) and spending time talking to family carers and support staff. Students often are initially surprised by this way of working.

In reality, I found one of the challenges of running a dysphagia placement in this setting was trying to fit in discussion time, as so much time is spent out in the community; car journeys became debriefing sessions and question times! It seemed that, with the focus being only on dysphagia, the students were less independent, spending most of their time shadowing speech and language therapists. Initially, I found it a challenge to strike a balance between observation and practical experience. However, once I'd given it some thought, there were adequate tasks the students could do with little or no supervision.

Adapting *The Dysphagia Placement Workbook* for this setting

I had the preconception that the workbook was mostly geared towards hospital-based placements, when in reality it worked very well in the Adults with Learning Disabilities (ALD) setting too. I found it worked to think of the workbook as a guide, and not to focus on the set activities as not all of them need to be completed. Some activities, such as standard bedside assessment, were not going to be possible in the community and I tried to arrange for the students to spend some time in our community hospital to experience this.

I believe that a placement that focuses on dysphagia in an ALD setting provides a holistic experience for students. Frequently, a variety of interesting and challenging issues occur, such as best interest decisions, safeguarding vulnerable adults, conflict of interests and cross agency working. This has meant that students actually move beyond the workbook goals, enabling them to think more widely and therefore offering a richer community experience.

Having the workbook was really useful, particularly as community work tends to be unpredictable, for example when there are last minute cancellations or changes. It was something that the students could get on with, and they didn't need to be with me all the time. It enabled them to self-direct their own learning and also helped me plan the placement. I tried to organize a week-long placement by initially trying to cover the workbook activities and then filled in the gaps with the other ideas I had, e.g. a visit to a day centre.

Tips for other clinicians

Think holistically

I really wanted the students to see that working with service users with learning disabilities is more than just a swallow observation, and that simply because the setting is not "medical" it doesn't mean that the dysphagia needs of the clients are not complex. Where possible, I encouraged students to attend 'best interest', safeguarding, end of life and professionals meetings. I also supported students to consider The Mental Capacity Act, 2005 and the impact on clinical decision making.

I tried to include PEG cases where service users were trialling small amounts of oral tastes, having oral care programmes as well as end stage dementia cases. Students were guided to think about keeping people safe as well as quality of life. This was to support their awareness of the realities of risk management and person-centred care.

Visit day centres

Wherever possible, students spent lunchtimes in a day centre for people with profound and multiple learning disabilities. This provided opportunities to observe a setting where most of the service users require some form of dysphagia management. Students were encouraged to reflect on issues around catering, pressure on support staff in relation to compliance with programmes, and risk management.

Screening

One of the real benefits for both the students and myself was encouraging them to carry out telephone screening for reviews. Initially, the students observed me complete one and then role played a review. They then required minimal support to complete screens independently. This was a great time saver for me. I tended to give them clients that I knew well so that I already had up-to-date knowledge for when they fed back.

Writing basic guidelines

After shadowing or jointly assessing clients, I asked students to fill in basic summary guidelines. I encouraged them to use templates and look at examples. This was good practice for them and also helped me in terms of time.

Taking case histories

The students were able to look through case files in detail and spend time completing case histories. Although we have our own case history forms, I asked the students to develop their own for specific cases, e.g. when reviewing a taster programme or talking to a support worker in a busy day centre.

MDT

Where possible, I arranged for the students to meet or shadow other relevant professional practitioners involved in dysphagia management, e.g. physiotherapists, dietitians, community nurses, etc.

Having two students together

I really found it much easier having two students. They could travel to various venues themselves, complete observations, discuss cases and articles together and also prepare resources jointly. Space can be an issue if you work in a small or busy office but there are always solutions to these problems!

Training

It is beneficial to run the placement to coincide with any training you may be planning. This was a good opportunity for the students I had on placement to have an introduction to dysphagia and ALD. Attending the training also gave the students a chance to liaise with carers, listen to discussions and understand some of the challenges carers face on a day-to-day basis.

Presentations

I asked the junior therapists to prepare short presentations on interesting cases, to explain their rationales and how they used evidence-based practice. They then presented these to the students followed by questions and discussion.

This was a good learning and development opportunity for both junior staff and students.

Formal teaching and discussion

It is a good idea to schedule in a couple of meetings on placement where you can offer some formal discussion or do some teaching. These meetings do not need to be long. I mostly used my own work from other training I had done. Some of the topics covered were: the normal swallow; signs and symptoms of risk; the free water protocol; pros and cons of thickeners, etc. I have been able to use these resources successfully with other students.

Key reading

It is worth getting the students to read key literature relevant to your clinical area. Discussion of this reading was beneficial, and we also got the students to contribute to the journal club if it occurred whilst they were on placement.

Mini projects

Setting mini-projects for students is another good learning experience. Short projects I have used include:

- Developing a consent form
- Making a poster about thickening fluids
- Putting together a leaflet about soft foods
- Looking for specific evidence to support an approach

They don't need to be with you all the time

The students really do not need constant supervision on this type of placement. Many of the activities in the workbook can be completed alone or with others. When the students were with me, they were able to lead on parts of the session as set out in the workbook, most notably the sections on case history taking, giving feedback, and so on.

Benefits

There are several benefits to offering a placement specifically focusing on dysphagia. It is intense, and the workbook provides structure and direction for both the clinician and students. If the placement is optional, as it was in my case, you find that the students have a real interest in dysphagia, which ensures motivation and a willingness to learn. All the students that I have had on placement have actively contributed to the service as a whole, for example by developing resources. The placement is a good way of raising awareness of dysphagia and learning disabilities as well as the complex ethical issues. I think that the students developed a new-found value and respect for this population as well as for community work.

3 Supporting Students in Clinical Writing

Naomi Cocks and Celia Harding
With contributions from Annie Aloysius, Nina Bharania, Stacey Lawrence, Camille Paynter and Emma Leach

When preparing to do any clinical writing, students and newly qualified therapists (NQTs) should be reminded of the three essential clinical writing preparation questions. These are:

1. Who is the audience?

2. What is the purpose?

3. What are the requirements?

Keeping these three things in mind will help them to ensure that their clinical writing has all the essential content and is structured in an appropriate manner.

The audience

The way in which notes, assessment findings and reports are written is very dependent on the setting. In some settings, all notes and reports are multidisciplinary; in other settings, more detailed speech and language therapy notes are also kept and separate speech and language therapy reports are written. Before a student attempts to undertake any clinical writing in your environment it is essential for them to be aware of the audience who will be reading it. Multidisciplinary notes and reports should be concise and written in a way that other professionals are able to understand. Referral reports to other speech and language therapy services should be detailed enough so that the speech and language therapist who is taking over can pick up the care and management of the client from where the referring clinician left off.

The purpose

When teaching students and NQTs how to write case notes, assessment findings and reports in your setting, it is essential to remind them of the purpose of case notes and reports. Case notes and reports have a number of functions including:

- Providing a legal record of events
- Documenting the effectiveness of treatment, including providing information about baseline assessments, management plan, and progress or decline
- Communicating with other speech and language therapists and professionals about assessment results and management, including prognosis, advice, precautions, recommendations for further assessment, likely next step in management and reasons for discharge.

These functions should always be kept in mind when writing case notes and reports.

One way of ensuring that all this essential content is included is to ask the student/NQT the following questions:

"If you could not come in to work tomorrow and no one could get in contact with you, would another therapist be able to pick up your notes and be able to know what has happened in the past with this client? Would they know what they should do in the next session with this client?"

"If in 3 years' time, these notes or this report were used in a legal case, would it be clear what happened with this client, what your clinical decisions were and why?"

The requirements

Students and NQTs should also be made aware of record keeping requirements for both the relevant facility and accreditation body (in Australia: Speech

Pathology Australia; in the UK: the Royal College of Speech and Language Therapists and the Health Professional Council).

Students should be made aware of requirements concerning:

- What content should be included in documentation

- When documentation should occur, e.g. within 24 hours for case notes

- Confidentiality, e.g. where notes and reports are kept and who is able to access them.

The structure and content

The structure and content of case notes and reports vary significantly between settings. It is helpful to show students and NQTs examples of notes and reports to ensure they have an understanding of what is expected in your setting.

Many speech and language therapists write problem-oriented medical records (POMR). The structure of POMR was first introduced by Weed in 1969, to help doctors to structure their medical notes. POMR are now more commonly known as 'SOAP notes'. The basic structure of SOAP notes are as follows: (S) subjective observations, (O) objective observations, (A) analysis of observations and (P) plan. In recent years, in addition to being used by doctors, the SOAP acronym has been used to aid other health professionals, including speech and language therapists, to structure their notes. It can be a useful framework, but often students and NQTs require more specific instructions about what to include in notes and in what order.

One way of ensuring that students and NQTs include all the essential content in their notes and reports is to provide them with a checklist. This also allows them to first check their own notes and reports before showing their clinical educator, which can be a useful timesaver. In the following pages you will find examples of checklists and of notes and reports in different settings. These checklists and examples can be shown to students and NQTs before undertaking some clinical writing to help them structure their clinical writing or shown to them afterwards in order to get them to reflect on their clinical writing abilities. These checklists and examples of clinical writing may not be appropriate for your setting and it may be more helpful if you create your own checklist.

Checklists for Case Note Entries

Checklist for Initial Assessment Case Note Entry

The following is a checklist that can be used for writing case notes for an initial assessment. Not all sections will be relevant for your setting or for all clients. You may wish to discuss which bits are and are not relevant in your setting with the student/NQT.

Put a tick in the box if you have included the following:

☐ Date of Assessment

☐ Time of Assessment

☐ Date of Referral

☐ Referral Source

☐ Reason for Referral

☐ Case History Information (to be included if not detailed by other professionals): including relevant medical history, medical diagnosis, whether previously seen by a speech and language therapist (when, why, outcome), highlight any relevant information detailed by other professionals that may be relevant for swallowing management, e.g. cognition, level of alertness

☐ Subjective observations: positioning, cognitive status, alertness

☐ Communication Assessment Results

☐ Details of how swallowing was assessed and the outcome of the swallowing assessment, including:

　☐ Results of oral musculature examination

　☐ Whether an oral trial was conducted – if not, why not

　☐ Consistencies of fluid or solids trials and whether there were any signs of aspiration/choking when trialling

　☐ Strategies/manoeuvres trialled and whether the strategies were effective

☐ Analysis of results, including:

    ☐ Aspiration risk

    ☐ Choking risk

☐ Plans and recommendations, including:

    ☐ Whether or not client should have oral intake

    ☐ Recommended fluid and/or solid consistencies

    ☐ Recommended strategies

    ☐ Recommended manoeuvres

    ☐ Prognosis

    ☐ When speech and language therapist plans to review

    ☐ Indicate whether client was involved in decision making

    ☐ Indicate whether strategies and plans have been communicated to client/family/other professionals

☐ Signature of Speech and Language Therapy Student with 'Speech and Language Therapy Student' written next to/underneath signature

☐ Signature of Clinical Educator with 'Speech and Language Therapist/Supervising Speech and Language Therapist/Speech and Language Therapist' written next to/underneath signature

☐ Pager/bleep number

Checklist for Review Assessment Case Note Entry

The following is a checklist that can be used for writing case notes for a review assessment. Not all sections will be relevant for your setting or all clients and this may be something that would be useful to discuss with the student/NQT.

Put a tick in the box if you have included the following:

☐ Date of Assessment

☐ Time of Assessment

- ☐ Reports from other health professionals/carer/client regarding the client's swallowing status, signs of aspiration, choking or pneumonia, e.g. the nurses report that client is managing diet well, nurses report no temperature spikes, medical team report regarding chest status

- ☐ Subjective observations: positioning, cognitive status, alertness

- ☐ Progress relating to communication

- ☐ Details of how swallowing was reassessed and the outcome of the swallowing assessment including:

  - ☐ Results of oral musculature examination

  - ☐ Whether an oral trial was conducted – if not, why not

  - ☐ Consistencies of fluid or solids trials and whether there were any signs of aspiration/choking when trialling

  - ☐ Strategies/manoeuvres trialled and whether the strategies were effective

- ☐ Analysis of results including:

  - ☐ Aspiration risk

  - ☐ Choking risk

- ☐ Plans and recommendations including:

  - ☐ Whether or not client should have oral intake

  - ☐ Recommended fluid and/or solid consistencies

  - ☐ Recommended strategies

  - ☐ Recommended manoeuvres

  - ☐ Prognosis

  - ☐ When speech and language therapist plans to review

  - ☐ Indicate whether client was involved in decision making

  - ☐ Indicate whether strategies and plan have been communicated to client/family/other professionals

- ☐ Signature of speech and language therapy student with 'Speech and Language Therapy Student' written next to/underneath signature

☐ Signature of Clinical Educator with 'Speech and Language Therapist/Supervising Speech and Language Therapist/Speech and Language Therapist' written next to/underneath signature

☐ Pager/bleep number

Examples of case note entries

The following are examples of case note entries. Examples have been selected from a range of clinical contexts.

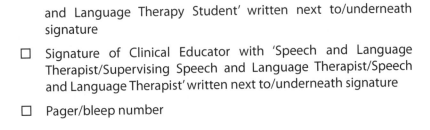

Adult Acute/Rehabilitation Hospital Setting

29/3/2011   12:30pm

Referral received from nursing on 28/3/2011 as client was coughing on thin fluids at lunch time.

Note client's history of stroke 10 years previously and diagnosis of dementia.

Assessment

The client was seated upright in bed and was alert. Client not oriented to time or place.

OME

Client unable to follow instructions and so unable to carry out a full OME. From observation no signs of facial or tongue weakness.

Oral Trial and Lunchtime Observation

Client able to feed and drink independently.

Trialled water: delayed onset of swallow, reduced hyoid elevation and coughing post swallow. Trialled level 1 nectar thick fluids: no coughing or voice change post-swallow. Trialled small soft diet lunch. Slightly extended duration of oral phase of swallow. No oral residue or pocketing post swallow. Client did not appear to have difficulties with chewing or swallowing the soft diet. Client finished small soft diet lunch and did not present with any difficulties with fatigue. No coughing observed for solids.

Analysis: Client at risk of aspiration when drinking thin fluids. No signs of risk of aspiration with level 1 nectar thick fluids. No signs of risks of choking or aspiration with soft diet.
Recommendations: Level 1 nectar thick fluids, soft diet, safe swallow strategies as outlined in care plan. Ongoing review from SLT appropriate. Current goals discussed and agreed with nursing team.
XXX, Speech and Language Therapist

27.06.2011 12.30

Aim: Swallow review
ATSP by OT following concern about swallow function during OT/PT session yesterday. Review of medical notes and discussion with nursing.
   Patient SOOB awake and alert. Cooperated with assessment.
Results:
Communication: Hypokinetic dysarthria characterized by decreased articulation, poor volume; exacerbated by decreased cognition and inability to follow cues and prompting.
Swallow: Wet vocal quality pre-assessment. Patient unable to initiate clearing swallow.
   Trialled water and observed with lunch. Pt able to self feed once set up. Oral phase: functional bolus co-ordination and transfer
Pharyngeal phase:
   – hyolaryngeal excursion palpated
   – nil overt delay in trigger
   – nil coughing during meal
   – occasional double swallows
   – fluctuating vocal quality - cleared during meals
Impression: Nil overt signs of aspiration during lunch observation; however, cannot rule out silent aspiration
   – swallow function likely to fluctuate due to a variety of factors: time of day; medication regime; cognition; medical status
   – VFSS will not inform ongoing management due to pt's fluctuating state, therefore more appropriate to manage based on clinical presentation

Rec:
  - continue normal diet
  - pt sitting out of bed for meals. Assistance with set up
  - regular SLT r/v during inpatient admission
Plan: refer to community SLT and PD clinic SLT and monitor in future
XXX, Speech and Language Therapist

26.06.2011 15.00
Speech and Language Therapy (Review)
Attended to review swallow
Review of medical notes and discussion with nursing staff: tolerating normal fluids and pureed diet. Chest clear. Obs stable.
  O/E: Pt SOOB. Alert and communicative. Recalling information from previous SLT r/v
  - SpO$_2$ >95%; RR18; Afebrile as charted
  - pt denying any difficulties with swallowing or coughing when eating and drinking
Swallow review: Trialled with bread, biscuit and water
  - prompt oral phase with fluids
  - adequate mastication and manipulation of solid bolus
  - adequate swallow trigger
  - mildly reduced laryngeal excursion with fluids
  - age appropriate with solids
  - 1–2 swallows to clear across consistencies (WNL)
  - no evidence of penetration or aspiration across consistencies
Imp: suitable for upgrade to normal diet
Recs:
  1. normal diet and fluids when alert and upright
  2. small mouthfuls
  3. pt to pace himself
  4. pt to avoid oral intake with SOB
Above strategies have been discussed with patient
Plan: to review 1/7. If tolerating upgrade, will discharge from SLT
XXX , Speech and Language Therapist

21.01.2011 16.00

Speech and Language Therapy

Thank you for referring this 82 year old woman admitted on 7.01.2011 with GI bleed and increased right sided weakness.

   O/E: Pt resting in bed. Niece Mandy present – she reported patient's daughter is on holiday and will return on Saturday.

Results:

Oromotor: Note cranial nerve assessment on admission was unimpaired

CNV: Functional jaw opening

CNVII: Right sided facial (lower quadrant) and lip weakness

CNIX-X-XI: Right soft palate weakness/asymmetry on phonation; weak voice when able to produce; pt unable to swallow to command; spontaneous swallows observed

CNXII: Limited tongue protusion on lateral movements – ax limited by decreased comprehension

Swallow:

Oral trials: 3 x sips water

Oral phase: appropriate lip contact with cup. Reduced bolus manipulation; poor a-p transfer

Pharyngeal phase: hyolaryngeal excursion palpated. Significant delay in pharyngeal swallow trigger; cough post swallow

Communication:

Comprehension

   – answering 'yes' to all questions

   – unreliable yes/no

   – unable to follow stage 1 commands

Verbal Expression

   – limited verbal expression – only used 'yes' and 'I think'

   – nil automatic speech – unable to count

   – unable to say name

Impression:

   • Oropharyngeal dysphagia with evidence of aspiration post-swallow

   • Receptive and expressive aphasia consistent with (L) CVA

   • (R) cranial nerve involvement (CNVII, CNIX and CNX) consistent with (L) UMN lesion

Rec:
- Oral intake contraindicated due to aspiration risk
- Team to consider alternative nutrition/hydration
- Team please consider communication impairment – patient significantly impaired receptively and expressively

Plan: SLT to R/V 1/7

XXX, Speech and Language Therapist

Adults with Learning Disability Community Setting

27/04/2011

Review telephone call

Following receiving monitoring charts, noted that consistent coughing on soft bite size with other signs of aspiration also, e.g. watery eyes, red complexion

On 20/4/2011 recommended downgrade to soft moist mash with a fork and to continue with normal fluids

Called today to review downgrade. Spoke with Sharon [key worker]. She reported that client much better, less coughing and other signs reduced

Asked Sharon to send over monitoring charts completed since change in texture modification

Action: Review charts, finalise guidelines, re observe if necessary

XXX, Speech and Language Therapist

21/02/2011

Telephone review completed with Home Manager Julie Simpson

Client last seen 6 months ago, recommended normal fluids and pureed meals

See telephone screen summary sheet (included in SLT section of MDT Health File) for full details

In summary:

2 chest infections, significant weight loss and occasional coughing (on foods and drinks) since last assessment

ACTION:

Booked breakfast time Ax 8am 24/02/2011

XXX, Speech and Language Therapist

24/02/2011

B'fast Ax, client supported by keyworker (Joe Bloggs)
Full Ax completed: see SLT section of MDT file for details
In summary client observed to be eating weetabix, and drinking tea
Limited oral movements observable, coughing, red face, watery eyes all visible, unable to observe laryngeal elevation when swallowing foods and drinks
Joe Bloggs reported that this is typical of mealtimes
ACTIONS:
Trial syrup thick fluids, advised and gave info re: smooth puree foods
Monitor x1 week
Contact hospital SLT to query whether possible to carry out VFSS
XXX, Speech and Language Therapist

13/04/2011

Dysphagia Ax at home 12.30pm
Referral received from Home Manager on 08/04/11 regarding increased coughing during mealtimes – see enclosed for referral and telephone triage
Client supported by Rosie, senior support worker
Medical Hx
No recent hospital admissions
1 recent chest infection, no other symptoms
No warning signs other than coughing reported
Asthmatic, hiatus hernia
Limited mobility, uses walker and/or wheelchair
Epilepsy, Downs Syndrome, query Dementia (known to memory clinic)
Oral Care
Dependent for oral care, can be challenging
Unable to carry out oral care ax, teeth appeared to be decayed
OBSERVATION:
Environment
Seated in dining room, lots of distractions with TV on loudly. Sat with 2 other service users.

Positioning

Seated in a chair, slumped and head very low to table.

Feet also hanging; not reaching floor

Communication

Mostly non verbal, echolalic, observed repeating 'lunch', 'egg', query comprehension

Eating

Observed to be eating (self feeds) egg mayonnaise sandwich with no crusts cut into small bite size pieces and a yogurt with pieces of strawberry

Has a few teeth, used either his teeth or lips to break off sandwich, anterior posterior tongue movement visible with some 'munching', laryngeal elevation also visible. Adequate lip seal throughout

Anterior posterior tongue movement visible when eating yoghurt, with observed laryngeal elevation and audible swallow

Some residue in mouth post swallow

Tends to overload mouth and eat quickly

Becomes distracted by environment; looking around the room and watching staff

Staff prompted him verbally and used gesture to prompt him to eat his lunch on 3 occasions during the meal

No immediate signs of aspiration observed

Drinking

Observed drinking tea from a standard mug, used both hands to hold mug

Achieved lip seal, no loss of bolus

Laryngeal elevation observed and audible swallow. Vocalised post swallow – no gurgling heard

No immediate signs of aspiration observed

NOTE: reported to be managing medications, currently in tablet form

POSSIBLE RISKS:

Aspiration pneumonia due to:

Poor oral care and dependent for oral care

Respiratory problems and limited mobility

Complex health condition

Several medications

Choking:

Low tone

Few teeth
Limited tongue movement
Limited chewing
Overloading
Aspiration:
No immediate signs observed but increase in coughing reported
One recent chest Ix, no UTIs or weight loss
ACTIONS:
1. Interim guidelines left and explained to staff team: Currently on soft moist bite size foods and normal fluids – no change to recommendation at present time. Advised re: better positioning – keep upright and stable base for feet, advised verbal prompts to eat more slowly and less overloading
2. Monitoring charts x 1 week to see if specific foods are problematic, review and see again as necessary
3. Dysphagia leaflet given

SLT to refer to special care dentistry regarding poor oral care, unable to access high street dentist
XXX, Speech and Language Therapist

Paediatric setting
00/00/11
13.30
Speech and Language Therapy Review
Purpose:
- Ongoing monitoring of breast feeding
- Ongoing monitoring of non-nutritive sucking programme during tube feeding
- Ongoing monitoring of risk
- Ongoing parent support through feeding and communication programme

Observation:
- Baby rouses and wakes for feeds regularly at approx. 3 hourly intervals
- Baby tires during feeds, @ 10–15 minutes into breast feeding

- Mother observed removing Baby from her nipple each time Baby paused
- Baby opens her mouth when touched to the side of her mouth
- On stimulation, Baby will bring her tongue forward, but ? slight pucker at tongue tip?
- Able to demonstrate short sequential suck bursts, up to 4, then pauses
- Tongue grooved, pink and healthy with lateral movement post stimulation
- No oral residue. Secretions managed competently
- Sucking pattern:

i) Non-nutritive suck: gagged on initial stimulation. Took four attempts to stimulate a burst of two sucks, then four suck bursts

ii) Nutritive suck: able to organize self onto the breast, then suck. Completed four sequential suck bursts, three–four sucks per burst. No significant jaw excursion. No gagging.

ACTION/GOALS DISCUSSED AND AGREED WITH MOTHER AND NURSE:

- Advised Mum not to keep removing nipple from Baby when she stops sucking. Discusses shaping the nipple rather to remove, and re-stimulating sucking
- On-going non-nutritive sucking programme for the first 10 minutes of a tube feed. Mum to stimulate three sequential suck bursts three times
- Mum to 'read' Baby's non-verbal signals during feeding. We discussed key signs; please see Baby's programme in the file
- We will continue to monitor

XXX, Speech and Language Therapist

Bleep:

00/00/11
Time: 13.30
Speech and Language Therapy Review
Out patient review of progress with Paediatrician
Mother and father present

Purpose:
- To review pharyngeal status and oral motor competence during a mealtime
- To discuss with X any issues she felt she may be having with eating and drinking

Sensation:
There are no hyper- or hypo-sensitivity issues at present

Positioning:
X uses supportive seating for table top activities. This was noted to be at an appropriate height

Equipment:
X had a soft mash meal, fruit juice with a straw and a yoghurt. X can feed herself independently

On examination:
X was able to manipulate the soft mash effectively. She managed this more in the left side of her oral cavity. It was noted that with food that had slightly increased soft lumps, X appeared to be more effortful with chewing. X informed the SLT that she finds using a straw effective with fluid intake

ACTION AGREED WITH PARENTS, X AND PAEDIATRICIAN
- At present, X's needs are met with a modified diet (soft mash/soft lumps)
- X commented that use of a straw was the most effective method of fluid intake as it enabled her to be as independent as possible. However, she did express that this was more challenging when she was tired. Use of a valved straw was recommended
- Three month review agreed

XXX, Speech and Language Therapist
Bleep

Checklist for an assessment for referral report from acute setting

The following is a very brief checklist that could be used to write a referral report for an adult client in an acute care setting. The report checklist was developed for a referral report to another speech and language therapy department, e.g. when client is being referred to a community team from an acute setting. The client only had swallowing difficulties with no additional communication or cognitive difficulties. Similar checklists could be developed for different settings, for clients with both communication and dysphagia and for different types of reports.

Tips for writing reports:

- Remember to use past tense.

- Try to include examples.

- Consider who will receive the report – if it is a non-Speech and Language Therapist, remember to define or describe all jargon and use examples.

- Where relevant, write source of information, e.g. nurse's report.

BACKGROUND INFORMATION

- ☐ Client information: name, age, address, contact details
- ☐ Date of report
- ☐ Medical history and reason for admission
- ☐ Date of referral/admission
- ☐ Who referred the client and why?
- ☐ If medical history prior to admission is commonly associated with dysphagia then describe the history of swallowing difficulty prior to admission, what diet and fluids they were on when they were referred, what strategies they were recommended prior to admission
- ☐ Length of stay in acute setting

COMMUNICATION

- ☐ Date of initial assessment
- ☐ Description of client's communication at initial assessment, including all aspects of communication, with strengths and difficulties
- ☐ Description of therapy given
- ☐ Outcomes of therapy
- ☐ Communication abilities at time of referral

DYSPHAGIA

- ☐ Date of initial assessment
- ☐ Description of the client's presenting swallowing difficulties at initial assessment
- ☐ State the diet and fluid recommendations that were given after the initial assessment and if/how these changed during admission
- ☐ Describe any strategies that aided the client's swallow while they were an inpatient and if/how these changed during admission
- ☐ Describe any direct therapy that was carried out to improve swallow function, e.g. the Masako Manoeuvre, the rationale for this therapy and whether there was any evidence that it was effective
- ☐ Results of the videofluoroscopic swallowing study
- ☐ Swallowing abilities at time of referral to community team

CONCLUSION/SUMMARY

☐   Provide a brief summary of the report

RECOMMENDATIONS

☐   State whether the client's swallow should continue to be monitored by the community speech and language therapy team

☐   State whether any direct therapy for communication or swallow should be carried out and why

☐   State whether any strategies were useful for communication

☐   State any recommendations regarding safe swallow strategies

☐   State any recommendations regarding diet and fluids

☐   TYPE AND SIGN YOUR NAME AND YOUR POSITION

Note: As a student your clinical educator will also need to countersign your report.

Examples of Reports

The following are a range of examples of reports that students may come across on placements.

Speech and Language Therapy Handover Report
Acute Setting

30 November 2011

Mrs Hilda Peters
32 Northampton Square
London, EC1V0HB
DOB: 23 January 1959

Background Details

Mrs Hilda Peters is a 52-year-old woman who was admitted to City University Hospital on 15/8/2011 with a mid-brain and pons haemorrhagic CVA. She deteriorated post admission and was admitted to ITU where a tracheostomy was inserted 19/08/2011 and removed October 2011. PEG was inserted 08/09/2006.

Past medical history includes uncontrolled hypertension.

Prior to the stroke Hilda was working full time as a GP. She was living with her husband, Albert, in a 2-storey house.

Assessment Results

Hilda presented as motivated and compliant during speech and language therapy sessions. She often presented as labile when faced with new people or activities. This reduced with exposure to the event.

Cognition

The Occupational Therapist reported that Hilda did not present with any cognitive difficulties when completing a CVA screening assessment. Hilda presented with excellent memory skills and was able to generate appropriate long-term therapy goals. A full neuropsychology assessment would be beneficial.

Language

Auditory comprehension: Not formally assessed. At the time of handover, Hilda was able to follow instructions without evidence of difficulty. She rarely required information repeated.

Verbal expression: Not formally assessed. Hilda's verbal communication has been noted to be syntactically correct in everyday conversations with no evidence of word-finding difficulties. At the time of handover, Hilda used an alphabet board to assist her communication with unfamiliar listeners without difficulty. No dysphasia is evident informally.

Written expression: Not formally assessed due to upper limb weakness.

Oromotor: During her hospital stay Hilda made significant improvements with regards to her oromotor function.
At the time of handover her level of function was as follows:

CNV: Mildly reduced strength

CNVII: Limited facial asymmetry. Mildly reduced range of lip movement and lip seal

CNIX-X: Mildly rough and hypernasal vocal quality. Reduced velopharyngeal competence evident on VFSS 21/11/2011

CNXII: Moderate–severely reduced tongue range and strength of movement. Decreased coordination of movement

Speech: Hilda presents with moderate dysarthria characterized by reduced coordination of voicing, hypernasality and reduced accuracy of articulation. This is consistent with site of lesion.

Hilda has been participating in individual speech therapy sessions 4 days a week and group therapy sessions once a week. At the time of handover her current speech goals included increasing accuracy of articulation, improving self monitoring skills, reducing rate of speech (pacing) and increasing voicing control.

Pragmatics: Hilda presented as polite and friendly both in 1:1 and group sessions. She displayed compassion for other patients and was often observed to say encouraging remarks. At times she required prompting for appropriate turn taking which may reflect some difficulties with inhibition.

Swallowing: At the time of writing this report, PEG remains in situ (inserted 08/09/2011).

A videofluoroscopy was conducted on 21/11/2011 which evidenced moderate oropharyngeal dysphagia characterized by poor bolus control resulting in early spillover of bolus from oral cavity into pharynx, extended oral phase, reduced velopharyngeal coordination (one episode of mild regurgitation), delayed initiation of swallow, and mildly reduced laryngeal excursion. Occasional penetration of fluid into airways was evident and mild pooling in valleculae and pyriform sinus. Good sensation evident as immediate cough triggered when material penetrated airway.

Hilda was placed on a puree diet with stage 2 (3 scoops per 200 mls) thickened fluids on 23/11/2011. She initially required encouragement due to decreased confidence with oral intake but this improved.

Recommendations

Hilda would benefit from ongoing intensive speech and language therapy to continue progress in the areas of dysphagia, speech and voice. She would also benefit from neuropsychological assessment in the future.

If you have any queries or concerns regarding Hilda's speech and language therapy input or this report please do not hesitate to contact me at the Speech and Language Therapy Department. Our telephone number is XXXXXX.

XXX, Speech and Language Therapist

Speech and Language Therapy Report
Adults with Learning Disability Community Setting

Direct Line:	xxxx xxx xxxxx	Address of LD Team
e-mail:	xxxx.xxxx@xxxx.nhs.uk	
web:	xxx.xxxx.xxx.xx	Tel
Date:	09/08/2010	Fax

Name: Jane Smith   **DOB:** 17/07/1943

Address: xx xxxxxxx xxxx, xxxxxxx, xxx xxxx

REASON FOR REFERRAL

Jane was referred on 09/07/2010 by Poppy Jones (support worker) due to coughing at mealtimes and history of chest infections.

BACKGROUND INFORMATION

Jane was not previously known to Speech & Language Therapy. Current concerns have been ongoing since March this year. She has been reported to cough during and after mealtimes and has episodes of 'chestiness', but with no diagnosis of chest infection, since February 2010. She has had no recent weight loss or urinary tract infections. At the time of referral she was on normal foods and fluids.

She has a pacemaker and in the past had a double hernia operation. She has a diagnosis of Downs Syndrome. She is not known to the memory clinic.

SUMMARY OF ASSESSMENT

Location:

Jane was assessed at home on 13/07/2010. She was supported by various members of staff including John and Sandra.

She was seated at the table in the kitchen on a standard dining chair with other staff and service users. Her feet were stable on the floor; however, her body was not in line and upright. She uses standard cutlery and crockery.

At rest she has an open mouth posture and protruding tongue. She communicates using nodding, vocalisations, facial expressions, body language and some single words.

Eating

She was observed to be eating beans on toast cut into quarters with small pieces of lettuce and cucumber in a dressing and finely chopped fruit salad mixed with cream.

Oral Stage: Able to achieve lip closure, broke down the toast into small pieces using a fork or fingers, no loss of bolus. Anterior posterior tongue movement observed, with some tongue thrust protrusion. Cheek muscle movement observed, with munching and rotary type jaw movement with some lateral jaw movements and anterior posterior thrusting. Seemed to be chewing although quite disorganized. Oral transit time seemed slow.

Pharyngeal Stage: Laryngeal elevation observed. Due to slow oral transit time (lots of oral movement and repetition of movement) swallow appeared delayed.

Overall: Ate approximately three quarters of the beans on toast and only a few spoons of the fruit salad. Tried one mouthful of the lettuce and cucumber and 'spat' back out after attempting to chew. No signs of aspiration during or immediately after eating.

Drinking

Jane was observed to be drinking orange squash from a glass.

Oral Stage: She achieved lip seal and there was no loss of liquid, oral transit time seemed normal.

Pharyngeal Stage: Laryngeal elevation was observed and swallow was audible, both observed consistently.

Overall: No signs of aspiration during or immediately after drinking.

Her home staff have also reviewed the consistency of all her medications, with support from SLT and the GP – see relevant correspondence.

Following interim recommendations (soft diet) Jane's staff team were given monitoring charts for one week, on review of these charts there was no record of any coughing or other warning signs of aspiration on any foods or drinks.

POSSIBLE AREAS OF RISK

Risk of aspiration pneumonia due to:

- Dependent for oral care
- Mouth/dental disease
- Bacteria in the mouth can be inhaled into the chest causing infection
- Declining mobility
- Reduced mobility indicates poor pulmonary clearance, making it difficult to fight infection, e.g. chest infection

Risk of asphyxiation (choking) due to:

- Low muscle tone
- No teeth
- Limited tongue movements and protruding tongue
- Limitations to chew function

Risk of aspiration:

- Reports of occasional coughing and sounding 'chesty'

RECOMMENDATIONS

Positioning:

- Jane should be seated in an upright position
- Her feet should have a stable base
- The table she eats from should be at an appropriate level
- She should be alert
- It is essential that Jane remains in good positioning as poor position will increase her risk of aspiration and choking

Drinks:

- Currently appears to be safe on normal fluids
- Should be monitored by staff for any changes

Foods:

- SOFT MOIST foods
- Small bite-size pieces or finely chopped if not very soft
- NO foods that are hard, stringy, crunchy, dry or chewy
- See table of soft foods foods for further detail
- Always check the consistency before serving

Equipment:

- No changes
- Standard cutlery and crockery

Assistance Required:

- Assistance to choose appropriate textured foods
- Assistance to chop food

Oral Hygiene:

- It is essential to maintain good oral hygiene as this will help reduce possible infection in the mouth and chest
- Please contact the SLT team should you require further information or support

Training/Referral:

- Information regarding Dysphagia awareness training given to Home Manager
- SLT has referred Jane to memory clinic via GP, for Dementia screening
- SLT has referred Jane to physiotherapy for advice regarding positioning and possible chest physiotherapy programme
- SLT has written to the GP to review the texture/consistency of medications

INTERVENTION PLAN

- Jane will be reviewed again in 3 months' time
- In the interim she can be referred to the service
- Please note that any increase in chest problems or diagnosed chest infection should be reported to SLT
- Staff should ensure she has a good oral care regime

Actions Required:

- Carers and staff to follow above recommendations
- Staff should contact SLT immediately if/when necessary according to the criteria below

Criteria for re-referral:

Any signs of aspiration during or immediately after eating and drinking (coughing, choking, watery eyes, flushed cheeks, discomfort, breathing difficulties), or long-term symptoms such as weight loss, chest infections, urine infections, respiratory problems and pneumonia.

If you see any of these signs please refer to Speech and Language Therapy at xxxxxx Learning Disabilities Service by completing a referral form or call on xxxx xxx xxxx.

If the coughing continues and/or the person looks distressed and is struggling to breathe and is choking (during eating/drinking/taking medication) follow your first aid protocol and call 999 or take them to A&E. It may be that she has aspirated; food or drink may have gone into the lungs and she will need immediate medical attention.

XXX, Speech and Language Therapist

Cc. Home/ GP/ File

Paediatric example 1

PAEDIATRIC SPEECH AND LANGUAGE THERAPY REPORT

J is a 9 year 10 month young boy who was referred for a swallowing assessment with videofluoroscopy by Dr X, Consultant Paediatrician, and DL, Speech and Language Therapist. His current Speech and Language Therapist is RB.

J was born prematurely at 26 weeks. He has a diagnosis of spastic quadriplegic cerebral palsy, epilepsy, learning disabilities and visual impairment. J has had an increase in vomiting recently and weight loss. He also had a recent hospital admission for severe constipation that affected his desire to eat. J is under the care of Dr L, Gastroenterology Consultant, in relation to these symptoms as well as queries of malabsorption which may also be contributing to his weight loss.

His mealtimes can take up to one hour and J often only eats small amounts, sometimes refusing to eat at all. Whilst J particularly enjoys sweet foods, he does not always enjoy all his eating and drinking experiences. His eating and drinking opportunities are carefully timed to fit in with physiotherapy stretches and time in his standing frame to avoid vomiting after eating.

He eats his meals at school in a supported seating system and attempts are currently being made for the provision of the same seating at home as Mum feels his position and head support are much better with more support. J eats a modified diet of smooth purees and drinks thickened fluids from an open cup. He takes one Ensure high calorie drink a day and half an Ensure yogurt and is under the care of the dietitian.

J is fully dependent on adults to feed him. He is reported to cough and choke at mealtimes. He wears hyoscine patches due to excessive drooling.

He sometimes sounds phlegmy and congested and this will make him vomit, he has one large vomit about once a month that tends to clear his chest, he also has a strong productive cough. He does not suffer from chest infections.

This feeding pattern, alongside his poor growth of late, has led to the request for a videofluoroscopy in order to assess whether a swallowing problem may be contributing to his current difficulties.

Videofluoroscopy

J was screened using a lateral view. He was positioned in his specialist buggy in an upright position with his head and neck in midline. His neck was in extension when he ate solids but in a more neutral position for his drink. He was fed by his mother. He took smooth puree of medium consistency from a spoon and drank fluids thickened to a pudding consistency from an open cup.

Puree

J was noted to have a protracted oral phase with limited tongue movements and poor control observed. He had difficulties manipulating and transporting the food to the back of his mouth in order to trigger a swallow and residue coated the base of his tongue. The swallow was triggered at the valleculae. Post swallow residue was observed in the valleculae and pyriform sinuses and multiple swallows were needed to clear the residue. Penetration of the airway to the level of the vocal cords was observed. There was no cough. A small amount of silent aspiration was noted during the swallow.

Thickened Fluids

Head and neck position for liquid swallows was more flexed to 90 degrees. There was anterior spillage of fluids from his lips as a result of poor lip closure and oral control and usually when drinking he is assisted with jaw support. The swallow was triggered at the level of the valleculae. There was some residue seen in the valleculae and pyriform sinuses. No penetration or aspiration was observed.

Stridor was audible after the small amount of food and drink taken in the clinic. This may correlate with residue or the small amounts of airway penetration and aspiration. During and after eating J was noted to have a strong productive cough. This cough may be sufficient in expectorating and clearing the small amounts of food aspirated.

Summary and Recommendations

J presents with significant feeding and swallowing difficulties including risk of aspiration. In addition, he is having difficulties maintaining his growth and nutrition. Whilst not solely an outcome of poor oral feeding, extended length of mealtimes and reduced amounts are likely to be contributing to this.

These findings were discussed with J's mother. The following recommendations were also discussed:

- J would benefit from consideration of supplemental enteral feeding alongside oral feeding. This may help to optimize his growth and nutrition as well as reducing the risk of aspiration.

- J's oral control and swallow was noted to be better when positioned with his head and neck in a neutral position. He would benefit from ongoing support at school and home for specialist seating support and optimal positioning for mealtimes.

J will require ongoing support from his local Speech and Language Therapist in order to facilitate the recommendations made as a result of today's assessment.

Please contact me if you require any additional information.

XXX, Speech and Language Therapist

Paediatric example 2

ANOTHER HOSPITAL
To: Ms C S
Paediatric Speech and Language Therapist
X Community Hospital
Dear C S

Re : Baby D DoB: 10/10/10

Known problems:

- Born at 41 weeks – birth weight 4.2 kg

- Meconium aspiration

- Hypoxic ischemic encephalopathy (some brain stem injury noted)

- On ICU for 14 days

- Ventilation required for 11 days

- Persistent pulmonary hypertension

- Cardiorespiratory arrest

- Initially very hypotonic

I recently assessed Baby D at X Hospital on 15/10/10 prior to her discharge from their NNU. I wish to refer her to your Team. My initial assessment findings are as follows:

- Baby D had a nasogastric tube in place and no oral feeding had been attempted.

- I assessed Baby D's non-nutritive skills; her manangement of her own oral secretions was competent, and she was able to demonstrate a rythmic non-nutritive suck pattern. However, I did note that she needed at least three attempts of stimulating the tongue to enable her to produce a suck. Baby D's tongue was pink, grooved and healthy. Left sided tongue movement was slightly more competent than the right side, but it was judged that there was sufficient movement to produce some functional sucking skills. No facial or oral sensitivity difficulties were evident.

- Intra-oral pressure was variable, but with more stimulation using the pacifier a noted improvement during the assessment was noted.

- No changes in saturation levels or heart rate was noted during this assessment.

- An initial trial of 40 mls was attempted. A NUK vented medium flow rubber teat was used. Baby D needed an initial stimulation orally with a pacifier to enable her to position her tongue effectively for sucking; she still has a disorganized presentation when first stimulating the tongue. Then the bottle teat was placed in her mouth. Baby D demonstrated a 1:1 suck swallow pattern.

- Baby D did not tire, nor did she show any signs of saturation decreases or changes in heart rate. In addition, she was able to complete the 40 mls in 10 minutes. A further 40 mls was given. There were no excess sounds on laryngeal auscultation. Baby D will need careful winding during feeding and also pacing to ensure safety due to her previous history and difficulties.

- Baby D is able to breast feed and bottle feed safely. She has been at home for a week, and no risk signs have been evident. I plan to monior her at X hospital until you can pick up her case. I think that she is likely to have long-term communication needs as well as requiring feeding support and monitoring. I am happy to do a joint handover session here if that would be helpful.

Many thanks, all best wishes,

XX Speech and Language Therapist

Cc GP
Early Years Education Team
Paediatric Physiotherapist
Paediatric OT
File

Paediatric example 3

A N OTHER HOSPITAL

To: D W, Speech and Language Therapist
X Health Centre
Dear D W

Re: B C DOB: 03/05/07

It was very helpful to catch up with you today regarding B C. I am just writing to formally declare that I will now hand her intervention management back to you, and discharge her from the A N Other Hospital Caseload. I will discuss management of her swallowing shortly, but wanted to summarize her progress to date:

- B C had a VFSS on 09.03.10. This indicated direct aspiration with thin fluids. Thickener for fluids was immediately prescribed, and there have been no reported choking or aspiration episodes since this time. Fluids are thickened to a puree consistency. Her progress with managing normal food textures has been excellent, and she is able to manage her meals at home safely and with good functional skills. B C likes to feed herself using utensils as well as finger feeding independent of an adult.

- B C's attention and listening skills have steadily improved since she was initially seen. She responds well to boundaries and visual cues to support her. She is greatly supported when an adult uses simplified language, repetition, gesture as well as visual and verbal modelling.

- B C has always had a concrete grasp of her home routine and familiar routine commands within this context. She has extended her knowledge to include more abstract and complex information. She can cope with [two ICW] commands, [functional descriptions], [mixed name commands], as well as location of items across the room. She may still need repetition and visual prompting in these tasks. [Question distinction] ability is emerging, but further consolidation may be needed to prepare her for the increased demands of a nursery setting in the future. Early concept development has recently become apparent, with a clearer development and confidence with [verb knowledge] and [negation].

- Expressively, B C has always demonstrated appropriate communicative intent. She enjoys interaction opportunities with both adults and peers. She has a developing noun and verb vocabulary that is continuing. It is felt that her confidence band expressively is at the two clause level, although she may be capable of longer utterances when confident. She still echoes many phrases, but also rehearses them as if consolidating the vocabulary. Similarly, she does use chunked phrases.

I feel that B C is still showing a receptive and expressive delay, although she has undoubtedly made excellent progress in all areas of her communication development. As she is now **not** going to transfer to the Child Development Team as was first indicated, I feel that her communication needs will best be met under your care. It may be that she will have the opportunity for some language and communication group work which I feel would greatly enhance her communicative competence.

B C will still need to have her use of thickener monitored, but I will be happy to evaluate her progress with this with you. Please do feel free to call me or e-mail me at any time should you want to discuss B C with me.

Many thanks, and all good wishes,

Yours sincerely,

XXX

Speech and Language Therapist

Paediatric example 4

Videofluoroscopy Report

Name:

A Videofluoroscopic Swallow Study (VFSS) for E was requested by Dr R, Consultant Community Paediatrician, on the advice of Dr T , Consultant Paediatrician, Tertiary Hospital. The referral was redirected from X Tertiary Hospital to Y Tertiary Hospital after E became known to the Speech and Language Therapy team here during a recent hospital admission.

The referral was made to assess her swallowing in light of poor oral feeding, repeated hospital admissions due to pneumonia and chest infections and faltering growth.

E attended a feeding assessment with Videofluoroscopy today with her parents, local Occupational Therapist, BS, and local Speech and Language Therapist, OM.

E is a 4 year 3 month old girl who was born prematurely at 26 weeks gestation. She has diagnoses of chronic lung disease of prematurity, Dystonic/Athetoid Cerebral Palsy, Gastro-oesophageal Reflux Disease, and constipation.

Following a Paediatric Intensive Care admission in December 2009 for pneumonia, she was discharged home with supplementary nasogastric tube feeding as she was felt to be too weak and her respiratory health too compromised to maintain all her nutritional requirements orally.

She returned to full oral feeding two weeks ago albeit on a modified diet of soft lumpy and smooth purees. Prior to her admission in December 2009, she had been offered table foods of a chopped consistency at mealtimes.

At home E drinks thin fluids and Nutrini high energy milk from a Dr Brown bottle. She is usually positioned in her specialist supportive seating for main meals and is well supported on her parent's lap for snacks.

At school she drinks fluids or smoothies of a custard thickness from an open flexi-cup. She is positioned in her specialist supportive seating system for foods and drinks.

E is under the care of a local dietitian, although she has not been reviewed regularly. She takes 250 mls of Nutrini high energy formula per day to support her growth.

E's parents find it challenging to feed E and they appreciate that she may have some difficulties with her swallowing. In school she takes up to an hour to feed and often this impacts on time which could be spent socialising or in lessons. She fatigues throughout her mealtimes and is reported to expend a lot of energy eating.

Videofluoroscopic Swallowing Study

Consistencies attempted

Omnipaque was mixed with the following consistencies: smooth yoghurt, blackcurrant juice thickened to a custard consistency and blackcurrant juice unthickened. Thickened fluids were taken from an open flexi-cup and thin fluids from a bottle.

Positioning

E was unable to be screened in her usual supportive seating system as it has a metal head rest which makes it unsuitable for use in X-ray. A tumble form chair was not trialled as her local Occupational Therapist felt that her position would be so poor it would be unrepresentative of her normal seating positioning and would therefore be likely to have a significant negative impact on oral motor and swallow function. A corner seat was explored; however, the radiographer was unable to screen laterally in this position.

With the agreement of the Consultant Radiologist and Radiographers and the wish and consent of E's father, E was screened in an upright position on his lap with additional head support offered by the Occupational Therapist. This position was not optimal.

Results

(Lateral View)

Oral stage: E demonstrated poor oral control, including bolus formation and transportation for all consistencies trialled. She had residue in her oral cavity post swallow for purees and thin fluids. Passive overspill over the base of the tongue to the valleculae and pyriform sinuses was observed on pureed textures.

Pharyngeal Stage:

Puree: All swallows were delayed with most triggering at the pyriform sinuses. There was residue in the oro-pharynx and pyrifom sinuses post swallows. One episode of silent aspiration was observed, which occurred during the swallow.

Thickened fluids: Swallows were triggered at the level of the valleculae. There was no residue noted post swallows. No laryngeal penetration/ aspiration noted.

Thin fluids: All swallows were delayed to the level of the pyriform sinuses. There was residue in the pharynx post swallow with noticeable pooling in the pyriform sinuses. E was noted to have one coughing episode post swallow during which she turned her head resulting in a loss of image. This may have been due to penetration or aspiration but cannot be judged.

E moved considerably throughout the assessment, notably during and post swallows which led to recurrent loss of image and possible missed episodes of laryngeal penetration or aspiration.

Oesophageal Stage: *Not assessed on this occasion*

Summary and Recommendations

In view of the above results alongside clinical presentation and history, E is considered to present as high risk of aspiration for both purees and thin liquids. She may be safe to take small amounts orally for pleasure; however, she is likely to be unable to safely manage the required intake needed for adequate nutrition, hydration and growth. This is in part due to the poor oral control demonstrated, which is clearly impacting on feeding efficiency, evidenced by protracted mealtimes and fatigue.

These results were discussed with E's parents alongside her local Speech and Language Therapist and Occupational Therapist. The following recommendations were made:

- E would benefit from consideration of a gastrostomy to supplement small amounts of oral feeding. This will reduce the risk of aspiration and support her in order to optimize her growth and development.

- E should take her fluids thickened to a custard consistency from a flexi-cup. Thickened fluids were swallowed efficiently today. Cessation of the use of a bottle may reduce immature patterns of tongue movement and, as a result, provide increased oral control for all textures. This will require ongoing support from her local Speech and Language Therapist.

- Removing bottle drinking from E's routine may impact on her hydration as she may not be able to drink the equivalent fluid amounts over the day. NG tube feeding was discussed as a short-term option to support her nutritional and hydration requirements, but is felt to be unmanageable for her parents. It may therefore mean that some bottle drinking is required despite the aspiration risk.

- E would benefit from more regular ongoing dietetic support in order to advise and support her weight and growth. Dietary support in the form of high calorie/energy food and drinks may enable her parents to reduce the volumes she needs to take orally and therefore reduce frequency and/or length of time eating.

- Given E's weakened chest status and significant aspiration risk, she would benefit from a referral to the Respiratory/Dysphagia Clinic at X Tertiary Hospital. This referral can be made locally by her Community Paediatrician, Dr R. I would be happy for this report to support the referral.

- It was discussed that more challenging consistencies such as chopped foods, cakes and biscuits are likely to be more difficult for E to manage orally. This may as a result impact on her swallowing function – although this was not assessed today. Re-introduction of these consistencies should be explored in conjunction with E's local Speech and Language Therapist.

Kindly contact me for any additional information you may require.

XX Speech and Language Therapist

Glossary of Terms

Aspiration: Food, liquid or saliva entering the airway (trachea)

Penetration: Food, liquid or saliva penetrating to just above the level of the vocal folds, but not entering the airway (i.e. clearing; not aspirated)

Residue: The presence of food or liquid in the pharynx after swallowing

Reflux: The backward movement of food or liquid as in the case of Gastroesophageal reflux (GOR) or nasopharyngeal reflux

Cc GP, HV, File

Reference

Weed, L.L. (1969) Medical records, medical education, and patient care. The problem-oriented record as a basic tool. Cleveland, OH: Case Western Reserve University.

4 Case History Taking Templates

Naomi Cocks, Celia Harding, Nina Bharania, Annie Aloysius, Lesley Baker and Stacey Lawrence

In this chapter, we have included copies of templates for case history taking. They are designed to be used when conducting case history interviews with clients, carers, and/or other professionals. Some aspects of these examples can be used when gaining important information from the client's medical notes. These checklists can be shown to students/newly-qualified therapists (NQTs) or adapted so that they are more suited to the setting. They are designed to be used to support students/NQTs to complete Activity 3: Information Gathering in *The Dysphagia Placement Workbook*. Clinical Educators can also discuss with students/NQTs how the examples differ from those in use in their setting.

Paediatric examples

Neonatal Feeding Assessment

Date/time of assessment: SLT initials:	
Child's name:	**Birth weight:**
D.O.B.:	**Gestation at birth:**
Referrer/reported feeding problems:	**Corrected gestation/age:**

Prenatal History:

Family history:

Maternal health:

Pregnancy:

Perinatal/Birth History:

SVD/ECS/EMCS/other:

Apgars: 1   5   10

Neurological History:

Cranial ultrasound: MRI:

Tone/Handling: Medical neuro exam:

GI History:

Current weight/growth

Establishment of enteral feeds

TPN: OGT: NGT: Oral feeds:

Toleration of feeds:

Vomiting/GOR:

Respiratory History:

Intubation: Ventilation: CPAP: NPO2:   SVOA:

Respiratory rate at rest: O2 Sats at rest:

Cardiac History:

PDA   ASD/VSD/other: HR at rest:

Other:

Metabolic/sepsis/jaundice, etc

Medications

Feeding Chart Summary:	Mls/kg Schedule/hr:
Feeding intention: breast/bottle	Formula/MEBM/DEBM:
Lactation (24hr volumes/expression)	Breast/bottle/NGT/other:

Carer's description of feeding

Volume taken/duration:

Behaviours/concerns

Feeding Questionnaire – Parent/Carer Report

Some teams may devise specific questionnaires or case history templates to gain caseload specific information. Questions may be accompanied by a form of rating scale so that changes between appointments or between bouts of treatment may be evaluated. For example, a paediatric speech and language therapy team that assesses children with complex motor disorders prior to having an Intrathecal Baclofen (ITB) pump or Deep Brain Stimulation (DBS) surgery may wish to focus on asking parents and carers specific questions as follows:

- General health and any eating and drinking issues, including chest infections in recent weeks, and any challenges in managing to take medication orally
- Current eating, drinking and medicine regime including alternative feeding intake
- Environmental aspects of the mealtime, including positioning
- Time spent on mealtimes
- Amount taken with detailed reference to fluid intake
- Types of foods and drinks taken
- An evaluation of how many times, if at all, the child coughs, chokes or gags during a meal
- An evaluation of any episodes of pain and discomfort during or immediately after meals
- Identification of any specific challenging behaviours during meals and when they occur
- An evaluation of the ease with which the child feeds themselves
- An evaluation of the child's engagement with the meal
- An evaluation from the parent/carer of their feelings during the meal process
- A consideration of how the child eats in social contexts outside of the home environment

- A question about DBS/ITB surgery or change of medicine regime for the child with complex motor needs and the impact (if any) on eating and drinking immediately after surgery/changes and after a prolonged period

Adult Examples

Case History Information Template Acute Setting
Can be used to collect information from case notes, nursing staff and/or client themselves

Date of Admission:

Reason for Admission:

Date of Referral:

Source of Referral:

Reason for Referral:

Medical History (highlighting important and relevant medical history, e.g. neurological, gastro-oesophageal disorders, etc.):

Previous Speech and Language Therapy involvement:

Current medications and possible impact on swallow:

Any recent changes in medications or health that may have results in a change of swallow status:

Communication/cognitive status:

Level of alertness:

Any dietary considerations (e.g. diabetes, allergies):

Pre-admission diet and fluids:

Pre-admission method of nutritional intake and level of independence in feeding:

Current diet and fluids:

Current method of nutritional intake and level of independence in feeding:

Have there been any recent signs of aspiration and/or choking? If so, what were they? Coughing/gurgly voice/red face/feeling of food stuck/feeling of choking:

Does the client drool?

Does the client have difficulties keeping food in mouth?

Does the client have difficulties chewing? Is the difficulty affected by consistency?

Has speed of eating been affected? Faster/slower?

Is there food left in mouth after swallowing? Where does it catch?

Are multiple swallows required?

Has the client had any recent chest infections?

Do difficulties occur for all meals or is it more difficult for particular meals? Which meal is most difficult?

Speech and Language Therapy, Adult Learning Disabilities Service Dysphagia TRIAGE/CASE HISTORY

Adapted from the Central London Community Healthcare – Barnet Learning Disabilities Service Case History Form developed by Nina Bharania

---

Date referral received: Name of SLT:

Name of referrer: Name of carer completing screen:

1. Have they had any previous Dysphagia input/recommendation in place?

2. What are your main concerns about the person's eating and drinking?

3. What consistency of food/drink is the person currently on?

4. What is the person's diagnosis if any? (Dementia, epilepsy, CP, DC, ASD, etc)

5. Is the person PEG fed? If so, for how long and why was it fitted? Are they on tasters/oral intake?

6. For how long have the E&D difficulties described been going on?

7. Have you observed the person coughing during or after mealtimes (on food or drinks)?

8. Has the person had any recent choking episodes, when, on what? (query cramming, distractibility/alertness, chewing skills, etc)

9. Does the person display/have you observed (during or after eating and drinking)

    a. Watery/wet eyes

    b. Gurgly voice

    c. Change in complexion

10. Has the person had any chest infections within the last year? If so, when? Does the person sound chesty or gurgly?

11. Does the person have any sensory problems?

12. How is their general health (spiking temperature, changes in health, any illness, etc.)?

13. Is there any respiratory diagnosis?

14. Has the person lost weight? If so, how much? Was this intentional?

15. Has the person had any urinary tract infections recently?

16. Does the person have reflux? Do they ever regurgitate food?

17. Has the person been refusing foods or drinks? Are they getting enough fluids?

18. What medications is the person on? (think if texture modification)

19. Are there any difficulties with oral care (ask them to describe, ask about dentition)

20. Does the person have a physical disability? What is the diagnosis?

Mobility	**Independent**		☐
	Limited mobility/uses aid		☐
	Wheelchair dependent		☐
	Special seating		☐
	Standard seating		☐
Scoliosis	Moderate	☐	
	Severe	☐	
Kyphosis	Moderate	☐	
	Severe	☐	

21. Has the person been admitted to hospital recently? If so what was it for?

CONCLUSIONS

URGENT	Y/N	NON URGENT	Y/N
Current (aspiration) pneumonia		Food refusal	
History of (aspiration) pneumonia		Oral stage problems, e.g. loss of food from mouth	
Current chest infections		Behavioural difficulties at mealtimes	
History of chest infections		Fast eating	
History of serious choking (e.g. hospital/paramedics)		Occasional coughing when eating/drinking	
Coughing at every meal/every drink		Gradual weight loss	
Sudden weight loss		Long mealtimes	
BMI <15		Difficulty feeding self	
Sudden change in eating/ drinking skills		General advice	
Respiratory distress when eating/drinking		UTI	

5 Information about the DVD and How to Use It

Naomi Cocks and Celia Harding
With contributions from Camille Paynter

The DVD

The DVD that is included in this book has been designed to be used to enhance activities in *The Dysphagia Placement Workbook*, in teaching/discussion sessions and in self-directed learning activities. It consists of three sections:

- Thickened Fluids
- Oral Motor Examination and Swallow Screen
- Videofluoroscopic Swallowing Study

These will each be discussed separately.

Thickened Fluids

This section of the DVD includes a demonstration of how to make thickened fluids. It is designed to be used alongside Activity 11 of *The Dysphagia Placement Workbook*. In Activity 11, students/newly-qualified therapists (NQTs) are encouraged to read and reflect on a number of resources. These include: research on the evidence for prescribing thickened fluids in dysphagia management; articles which discuss some of the issues and limitations of using thickened fluids; and the guidelines for using thickened fluids. Students/NQTs are then encouraged to make some thickened fluid, to trial the fluid and to reflect on the difficulties associated with making and taking thickened fluids. This section of the DVD could be shown to students/NQTs prior to them making thickened fluids. It is important to highlight to students/NQTs that the instructions on how to make thickened fluids depend on the brand of thickened fluids and that they should consult the instructions relevant to the brand used at their setting before attempting to make thickened fluids.

The DVD could also be used to stimulate discussion of the following topics:

- When do you prescribe thickened fluids?

- What are the advantages/disadvantages of prescribing thickened fluids?

- What do you need to think about when deciding which brand of thickened fluids to use (consider starch vs gum-based thickener, pre-thickened vs not pre-thickened, cost, taste, allergies, sugar content, etc)?

Additional activities associated with making thickened fluids that NQTs/ students could be asked to do include:

- Making handouts for carers/clients/catering staff with instructions on how to make different levels of thickened fluids.

- Providing training to catering staff/carers on how to make thickened fluids.

- Carrying out an audit of viscosity of thickened fluids in your setting.

Oral Motor Examination and Swallow Screen

This section of the DVD includes a demonstration of a basic oral motor examination (OME) and swallow screen. It represents the typical type of assessment that clinical educators may perform in the workplace.

This section of the DVD is designed to be used when students/NQTs are doing Activities 4 and 5 of *The Dysphagia Placement Workbook*. In these activities, students/NQTs role play carrying out an OME and oral trial with their peer before carrying out an OME and oral trial with a real client. This section of the DVD could be shown to students/NQTs as a model of an OME/ swallow screen before they do the role play. It is important to note that this is just one example of a basic OME and swallow screen protocol. Research suggests that the components of the OME and swallow screen vary between clinicians and settings (Martino, Pron, & Diamant, 2004; Mathers-Scmidt & Kurlinski, 2003; McCullogh, Wertz, Rosenbek, & Dinneen, 1999).

Some discussion topics that you could use with students/NQTs include:

- Think about how the OME and swallow screen differ in your setting. Why does it differ?

- When is an OME and swallow screen not appropriate?

- Think about what is being assessed in each component of the OME and swallow screen and why this is important. Students may wish to reflect on the differences between upper motor and lower motor neuron features that would be identified and differentiated during examination. There is some information on the video about what is being assessed; however, due to limited space for subtitles on the video screen a number of areas are not listed. For example, when a client opens their mouth, the clinician should be looking at the state of oral health, any physical abnormalities, dentition, xerostomia, etc., not just soft palate elevation which is included in the subtitle on the screen.

- Think about how it could be adapted for use with different populations, e.g. a patient with cognitive difficulties, a child with learning disability, etc., as well as reflecting on the different settings where such examinations would take place such as in a person's home, in a school, and so on.

Videofluoroscopic Swallowing Study

The Videofluoroscopic Swallowing Study (VFSS) section consists of:

- Preparing for a videofluoroscopic swallowing study

- Carrying out a videofluoroscopic swallowing study

- Videofluoroscopic swallowing study of an individual with a normal swallow

- Videofluoroscopic swallowing study of an elderly individual

- Videofluoroscopic swallowing study of an individual who aspirates

This section of the DVD can be used alongside Activity 8 in *The Dysphagia Placement Workbook*. In this activity, students/NQTs are encouraged to first read relevant articles and guidelines about VFSS before watching a VFSS. This section of the DVD has been included so that students/NQTs who are in settings in which they do not have access to VFSS can still complete this activity. All questions included in Activity 8 can be completed using the DVD without needing access to a VFSS suite. For question 1(c), in which students are asked to "…comment on how the VFSS findings compare to the outcomes of the bedside assessment. Do the VFSS findings contribute anything new?", students can be provided with the following community speech and language therapy entry:

10.5.2010 13:00 Swallowing Review

Lunchtime assessment in patient dining room.

Nursing and medical team notes indicate that since last review by SLT a week ago that client has been managing 1/2 portions of thick puree diet and syrup thick fluids with no difficulties and that there have been no signs of aspiration or choking. Chest remains clear with no signs of chest infection.

Assessment: Patient was seated upright in his wheelchair at the dining table and was alert. Pt reported that he had been doing his swallowing exercises regularly and that he had not been having any difficulties swallowing. He reported that he didn't like the thickened fluids. Pt was reminded why he had been prescribed thickened fluids.

Fluids: Oral trial of thin fluids Delayed initiation of swallow, reduced hyolaryngeal excursion, coughing post swallow. Trialled syrup consistency. Head extension used in an attempt to initiate swallow. Spontaneously double-swallowed. No coughing or wet voice post swallow.

Solids: Observed patient eating 1/2 portion thick puree lunch with dessert spoon. Patient had difficulties with the oral stage of the swallow. His oral stage was extended and he appeared to have difficulty manipulating the bolus. Mild oral residue in the mouth post swallow. Patient required prompting to clear. No coughing was observed post swallow. Patient became fatigued halfway through the meal and was unable to finish the 1/2 portion of thick puree meal.

Recommendations:

1. To continue with 1/2 puree diet and syrup thick fluids

2. Dietetics, please review client with regards to hydration and nutrition levels

SLT Plan:

    1. SLT to review pt with regards to swallowing exercises in 1/52

    2. To refer to City University London Hospital for VFSS review

XX Speech and Language Therapist

While the VFSSs on the DVD are designed to be used alongside Activity 8 in *The Dysphagia Placement Workbook*, they could also be used in other activities and to stimulate discussion. VFSS reports of the clients on the DVD have been included in this book to be used in the additional activities and to aid in the discussion of VFSS.

Other activities could include:

- Students/NQTs read the above notes and hypothesize what the client's VFSS might look like. After a discussion of the hypotheses, show the students the real VFSS.
- Students/NQTs could write mock VFSS reports for the clients on the DVD. They could then compare the reports they produced with the ones provided.

Students/NQTs could also be encouraged to discuss the following:

- the advantages and limitations of using VFSS in an assessment battery
- when you would use a VFSS and when you wouldn't
- how the swallow is affected by age
- what aspiration looks like
- what the next step would be in the management of the client who aspirates
- how a child's VFSS may look different
- how the VFSS of a client they have seen on placement would differ to the VFSS they have just watched on the DVD

Speech and Language Therapy Report for Videofluoroscopic Swallowing Study of a Normal Swallow

RELEVANT BACKGROUND AND MEDICAL HISTORY

Mrs Xxxx was referred for a videofluoroscopic swallowing study by her Consultant Chest Physician, Dr Xxx, to assess for aspiration due to four-year history of episodic paroxysmal coughing.

Mrs Xxxx attended VFSS clinic 29.6.11. Oromotor assessment was unremarkable. She reports occasional, intermittent 'lisping' that is noticed by her partner but not herself. No neurological past history is noted.

PURPOSE OF STUDY

1. TO ASSESS RISK OF ASPIRATION
2. TO EVALUATE SWALLOWING PHYSIOLOGY

SUMMARY OF RESULTS

Diagnosis: WITHIN NORMAL LIMITS

Description of the swallowing impairment: Mrs Xxxx presents with swallow function within normal limits.

DIET/FLUID RECOMMENDATIONS

Fluids: NORMAL CONSISTENCY

Diet: NORMAL

CLINICAL RECOMMENDATIONS

1. NONE
2. NONE

DESCRIPTION OF VIDEOFLUOROSCOPIC SWALLOWING STUDY

Positioning:	Independently sitting in chair		Imaging View:	Lateral
Consistencies Trialled:	Fluid: Omnipaque	Fed by: self	Bolus size (fluid): Unrestricted	
	Food: Solid	Fed by: self	Bolus size (food): Unrestricted	

Oral Phase:

- Nil abnormality detected
- Appropriate bolus coordination, cohesion and anterior–posterior propulsion was evident on fluid and solid consistencies.

Pharyngeal Phase:

- Nil abnormality detected
- Swallow triggered at base of tongue/valleculae (within normal limits for age)
- There was no evidence of airway penetration or aspiration on solid or liquid consistencies

Oesophageal Stage:

This was not assessed.

SUMMARY

Mrs Xxxx presents with swallow function within normal limits. There was no evidence of airway penetration or aspiration on solid or liquid consistencies

XX Speech and Language Therapist:

cc.

Report for Videofluoroscopic Swallowing Study of an Elderly Individual

SPEECH AND LANGUAGE THERAPY VIDEOFLUOROSCOPIC SWALLOWING STUDY REPORT

RELEVANT BACKGROUND AND MEDICAL HISTORY

Mrs X is an 81-year-old woman admitted to the City University London Hospital on 27/5/2011 with a three week history of general malaise and unresolving chest infection.

Significant past medical history includes oesophageal dysmotility (2009), brochiectasis (2008), ex-smoker. Mrs X reports a history of reflux and is taking PPI medication.

Mrs X denies swallowing difficulty but reports reflux of food. Bedside clinical assessment of swallow was unremarkable; however, a videofluoroscopic swallowing study was recommended to rule out silent aspiration.

PURPOSE OF STUDY

1. TO EVALUATE SWALLOWING PHYSIOLOGY
2. TO ASSESS FOR RISK OF SILENT ASPIRATION

SUMMARY OF RESULTS

DIAGNOSIS: WITHIN NORMAL LIMITS

DIET/FLUID RECOMMENDATIONS

FLUIDS: NORMAL CONSISTENCY

DIET: NORMAL DIET

CLINICAL RECOMMENDATIONS

1. Review of reflux

DESCRIPTION OF VIDEOFLUOROSCOPIC SWALLOWING STUDY

Positioning:	Seated in wheelchair	**Imaging View:**	Lateral	
Consistencies Trialled:	**Fluid:** Omnipaque (thin)	**Food:** Soft solid		
Fed by: Therapist	**Bolus size (fluid):** Sips		**Bolus size (food):** Teaspoon	

Oral Phase:

- Nil impairment; appropriate mastication and control of cohesive bolus for oral to pharyngeal transfer

Pharyngeal Phase:

- Valleculae filling prior to initiation of pharyngeal swallow which is age appropriate
- Nil pharyngeal residue post swallow
- Nil aspiration evident

Oesophageal Stage:

This was not assessed.

THERAPY RECOMMENDATIONS

None

SAFE SWALLOW RECOMMENDATIONS

None

SUMMARY

Mrs X presents with swallow function within age appropriate limits. She reports worsening reflux symptoms including reflux of food. Mrs X may benefit from a review of her medication or from gastroenterology.

XX Specialist Speech and Language Therapist

cc. Mrs X, SLT file, Medical notes, GP

Report for Videofluoroscopic Swallowing Study of a Patient who Aspirates

SPEECH AND LANGUAGE THERAPY VIDEOFLUOROSCOPIC SWALLOWING STUDY REPORT

Client's name: Mr X   DOB:

Address: SLT: XXXX

Hospital #:   Radiologist: XXXX

Date: 17.5.2011   Radiographer: XXXX

Referred by: Community SLT XXXX

RELEVANT BACKGROUND AND MEDICAL HISTORY

Mr X was referred for a videofluoroscopic swallowing study by his community speech and language therapist to assess whether he was suitable to be upgraded to a soft/moist diet (baseline consistency). Mr X had a posterior circulation infarct on 6/2/2011 which resulted in moderate–severe dysphagia, dysarthria and dysphonia. He was treated at the City University London Hospital. A videofluoroscopic swallowing study was performed on 16.2.2011. Following this he was recommended to have syrup thick fluids and a pureed diet. He was also recommended to commence swallow rehabilitation, specifically Shaker exercise, to target laryngeal excursion with the aim of improving cricopharyngeal opening.

Mr X's current speech and language therapist reported that he had been compliant with swallow rehabilitation. Mr X was also reported to have been tolerating previously recommended consistencies with no chest concerns.

Prior to his most recent CVA, Mr X had two previous CVAs in 2004 and 2009. His medical history also includes NIDDM and PVD.

The videofluoroscopic swallowing study was carried out on 17/5/2011 and was attended by his community speech and language therapist (Carrie Bradscore) and a nurse from City University London Nursing Home (John Preston). John reported that Mr X also has a PEG tube. He was unsure as to whether he was still receiving enteral feeding. John also reported that Mr X often fatigues during his meal and is unable to finish it.

PURPOSE OF STUDY

1. To evaluate swallowing physiology

2. For ongoing assessment and management of dysphagia

DESCRIPTION OF VIDEOFLUOROSCOPIC SWALLOWING STUDY

Baseline Oral Intake:	Pre CVA 2011 – normal fluids and a soft moist diet		
Pre-VFSS Intake:	Syrup thick fluids and a pureed diet		

Positioning:	Supported in wheelchair	Imaging View:	Lateral

Consistencies Trialled:	Fluid: Omnipaque (thin)	Fluid: Syrup thick fluid	Food: Smooth puree	Food: Soft moist (banana in angel delight)

Fed by: Therapist	Bolus size (fluid): Teaspoon	Bolus size (food): Teaspoon

Oral Phase:

- Adequate lip seal around spoon

- Poor control and containment (lingual to palatal contact) of fluid boli with premature spillage over the base of tongue into the pharynx

- Difficulty with posterior propulsion of pureed consistency with tongue pumping evident

- Incomplete mastication and breakdown of soft/moist consistency in addition to premature loss of this consistency into the pharynx

- Mild residue post swallow in the oral cavity observed to fall into the pharynx post swallow

- Of note, patient was observed to use head extension inconsistently in an attempt to assist posterior propulsion/initiation of the swallow

Pharyngeal Phase:

- Mild nasal regurgitation observed with fluids

- Swallow trigger variable across and within consistencies. With fluids, swallow generally triggered from pyriform sinus. Mild improvement to trigger with pureed consistency as the bolus overspills the epiglottic valleculae. Inconsistently delayed with soft moist consistency (on one bolus the pyriform sinus fills to capacity prior to initiation of swallow)

- Reduced laryngeal excursion resulting in incomplete epiglottic deflection and reduced cricopharyngeal opening. Duration of cricopharyngeal opening proving more problematic than degree of opening with regards to residue with the pyriform sinus

- Reduced base of tongue to posterior pharyngeal wall

approximation and pharyngeal contraction in addition to the above resulted in diffuse pharyngeal residue. This varied depending on the consistency, i.e. Normal fluids = mild diffuse residue. Syrup thick fluids (full teaspoon) = severe pyriform sinus residue, moderate epiglottic valleculae residue and base of tongue coating. Syrup thick fluids (1/2 teaspoon) = mild epiglottic valleculae residue only. Pureed consistency = variable. Mild-moderate epiglottic valleculae residue and base of tongue coating. Soft moist consistency = moderate epiglottic valleculae residue and mild pyriform sinus residue and base of tongue coating

- Spontaneous and prompted clearing swallows were effective in reducing pharyngeal residue

- Poor airway protection was observed with normal fluids with penetration and aspiration post swallow (on residue) and during and post swallow on the full teaspoon of syrup thick fluids. A reflexive cough was ineffective in clearing aspirated material with normal fluids. Aspiration of the full teaspoon of syrup thick fluids was silent. A prompted cough was not effective in clearing

- Penetration was observed with ½ teaspoon of syrup thick fluids; however, this appeared to be transient

- No direct aspiration was observed with pureed or soft moist consistency

- NB: direct assessment of penetration and aspiration was difficult post initial trial of fluids due to contrast seen within the laryngeal vestibule and subglottic space. A clinical correlation is therefore advised.

Oesophageal Stage:

Not directly assessed by speech and language therapy. Please refer to Radiology if concerned.

SUMMARY OF RESULTS

Diagnosis: MODERATE–SEVERE OROPHARYNGEAL DYSPHAGIA

Description of the swallowing impairment: Mr X presented with a moderate oropharyngeal dysphagia. The oral phase was characterized by poor oral control, containment and mastication which resulted in poor breakdown of solids, oral residue and premature spillage of consistencies into the pharynx. The pharyngeal phase was characterized by reduced velopharyngeal competence, a delayed swallow trigger, reduced laryngeal excursion and epiglottic inversion, poor pharyngeal contraction and incomplete airway protection. This resulted in mild nasal regurgitation with fluids, compromised airway prior to initiation of the swallow, diffuse pharyngeal residue and penetration and aspiration of certain consistencies. Airway response to aspiration was variable; however, reflexive and/or prompted coughing was ineffective in clearing aspirated materials. There was no aspiration evident with controlled bolus' size with syrup thick fluids and pureed consistency.

It was noted that this presentation was somewhat different from the previous videofluoroscopy. Clinical correlation was made at time of the assessment with the nurse present from the nursing home and the speech and language therapist present who reported that there had been no chest concerns since Mr X was commenced on modified consistencies in February.

RECOMMENDATIONS

It is recommended that Mr X continue with size controlled amounts of syrup thick fluids and a pureed diet with close monitoring of his chest. Should there be chest concerns, it is strongly recommended that further investigations be undertaken.

It is not suitable at this point in time for Mr X to be upgraded to a soft moist diet due to the incomplete mastication and breakdown of this consistency in addition to delayed swallow trigger compromising his airway.

It is recommended that Mr X continue his swallow rehabilitation with the Shaker Exercise. It is suggested that Mendelsohn's Manoeuvre also be incorporated targeting laryngeal excursion. In addition to this, Masako should be considered to improve base of tongue strength. A repeat videofluoroscopy is recommended in approximately 8 weeks' time to assess for further improvements.

DIET/FLUIDS
- 1. Fluids: ½ TEASPOON OF SYRUP THICK FLUIDS
- 2. Diet: PUREED DIET (BLENDED/LIQUIDIZED FOODS)

ADDITIONAL STRATEGIES/SAFE SWALLOW RECOMMENDATIONS

1. Give pureed consistency via a teaspoon
2. **Prompt a clearing swallow** if Mr X does not elicit one spontaneously
3. Discontinue eating and/or drinking if Mr X is coughing, his chest deteriorates or he experiences any difficulty breathing
4. Ensure Mr X is positioned upright and is alert for all oral intake (preferably sitting out in chair with 90 degree hip flexion)
5. Avoid distractions, e.g. turn off the radio or TV during meal times
6. **Crush medications** and give with **thickened fluids**. This recommendation was discussed with the City University London Hospital Pharmacist, Peter Brady, on 17.5.2011. He confirmed that crushing Mr X's medication and giving with thickened fluids would not result in any side effects or impact significantly on absorption.

CLINICAL RECOMMENDATIONS

1. Close monitoring of signs of aspiration
2. Ongoing speech and language therapy for dysphagia
3. Community speech and language therapist to discuss with community dietitian whether patient can receive top-up feeds and fluids via PEG in order to ensure patient receives adequate levels of nutrition and hydration.

XX Specialist Speech and Language Therapist
cc. Speech and Language Therapist, City University London Nursing Home
Dietician, City University London Nursing Home
SLT file
Medical notes

References

Martino, R., Pron, G., & Diamant, N. (2004) Oropharyngeal dysphagia: Surveying practice patterns of the speech and language pathologist. *Dysphagia, 19,* 165–176.

Mathers-Scmidt, B. & Kurlinski, M. (2003) Dysphagia evaluation practices: Inconsistencies in clinical assessment and instrumental examination decision-making. *Dysphagia, 18,* 114 125.

McCullogh, G.H., Wertz, R.T., Rosenbek, J.C., & Dinneen, C. (1999) Clinicians' preferences and practices in conducting clinical/bedside and videofluoroscopic swallowing examinations in an adult, neurogenic population. *American Journal of Speech Language Pathology, 8,* 149–163.

6 Additional Learning Activities and Projects

Naomi Cocks and Celia Harding

Introduction

While the workbook provides a range of activities that can support students and NQTs, as indicated by Nina in Chapter 2, it is also helpful to set a project to complete by students who are on placement. Such projects can result in something useful for the service, thus ensuring that students particularly 'give something back to the service'. Students can also work on these projects independently at quieter times during placement, or when clinical educators are busy.

Project suggestions

Developing handouts for carers and clients

In this project, students could develop a range of handouts to be given to carers or clients who have dysphagia. Students should be encouraged to think about research, think about how to explain complex concepts in simple terminology (e.g. what dysphagia is), and to evaluate what would be essential content and what could be left out. Thinking about the potential range of clients, including those who have comprehension or cognitive difficulties, could also be an essential part of this task.

An additional project might be to create handouts for children, for clients with specific communication difficulties or clients with learning disabilities. In these additional projects, students should be encouraged to think about how to present information so that it is most accessible for a client.

Some suggestions of handouts for clients and carers include the following:

1. A handout that explains what 'dysphagia' is.

2. A handout about what the speech and language therapy service does.

3. Instructions on how to thicken fluids to a particular thickness.

4. A handout that explains what a particular diet should and should not include, e.g. defining and focusing on a 'soft diet'.

5. A handout that explains what a VFSS or FEES assessment is, and how to prepare for it.

6. Instructions on how to carry out a specific swallow strategy or exercise.

7. General practice guidelines outlining safe swallow strategies.

Developing handouts and training resources for other professionals

In this project, students/NQTs could develop a range of resources which could be used for informing or training other professionals about dysphagia. In this task, students/NQTs should be encouraged to think about and research who the audience would be, what the audience is likely to know about the topic, how to explain certain concepts to this audience given their knowledge base, what essential content to include and how best to present material. By asking students to prepare the same materials for two different audiences, they may learn about different professional roles within the team and the level of knowledge and understanding of different professionals. This project could be adapted depending on the setting and the profession involved.

Some suggestions for training resources include:

1. A PowerPoint presentation that could be used in training other professionals, e.g. catering staff, nurses, health care assistants, teachers, etc.

2. Guidelines for when and how to refer to speech and language therapy services.

3. A handout on what dysphagia is and what a speech and language therapist does.

4. Instructions on how to thicken fluids to a particular thickness.

5. A handout that explains about what diet prescription should and should not include.

6. Instructions on how to carry out a specific swallowing strategy or exercise.

7. A handout on the importance of oral hygiene for a particular clinical group.

Quality monitoring

For this project, students would either develop a tool that can be used for monitoring the quality of a dysphagia service provided by a speech and language therapy or another service relating to dysphagia, e.g. catering services, or conduct a search for existing quality monitoring tools. If appropriate, the student may collect quality monitoring data with the tools.

Some suggested quality monitoring projects include:

1. Research the line spread test, and then use the line spread test to measure how thickened fluid changes over time, with temperature or with different drinks.

2. In an acute setting, research the line spread test and use this to determine whether all clients who have been prescribed a particular thickness (e.g. level 1 nectar thickness) are receiving drinks that are the same thickness. This may be carried out within one setting or across multiple settings.

3. Develop a form that can be used on a ward round at lunch time to collect statistics on whether clients are receiving the diet (e.g. soft diet) that they have been prescribed.

4. Design a small study in which thickened fluid wastage could be measured.

5. Design a questionnaire that can be given to a carer, client or other professional in order to gain feedback on dysphagia services.

6. Design a questionnaire that can be used to gain data concerning other professionals' knowledge of dysphagia before and after a training course.

7 Answers to the Pre-Placement Quizzes in *The Dysphagia Placement Workbook*

Celia Harding and Naomi Cocks

This chapter gives a general overview ᶜ the expected core elements essential to answering each pre-placement question. Where appropriate, clinical educators (CEs) may wish to elaborate further on some questions depending on the main focus of their clinical area. If students have not answered the questions correctly or comprehensively, it may be appropriate to direct them to the suggested references indicated. Where appropriate, we have given the relevant sections/page numbers of the following texts:

- Cichero, J. & Murdoch, B. (Eds) (2006) *Dysphagia: Foundation, theory and practice.* Chichester: John Wiley and Sons Ltd.

- Groher, M. & Crary, M. (2010) *Dysphagia: Clinical management in adults and children.* Missouri: Mosby.

- Daniels, S.D. & Huckabee, M.L. (2008) *Dysphagia following stroke.* Plural Publishing: San Diego.

- Logemann, J.A. (1998) *Evaluation and treatment of swallowing disorders.* Austin: Pro-Ed Publishers.

- Winstock, A. (2005) *Eating and drinking difficulties in children: A guide for practitioners.* Milton Keynes: Speechmark.

Pre-placement Quiz 1:
Dysphagia knowledge self-assessment answers

The answers to Quiz 1 in the accompanying book

- Cocks, N. & Harding, C. (2011) *The Dysphagia Placement Workbook.* London: J&R Press.

Instructions

1. Fill in the following table indicating the general functions of each of these cranial nerves, the impact that damage to the nerve will have on swallowing and how you test the function of the nerve.

Cranial nerve	General function	Impact of damage on swallowing	How the function of the nerve is tested
V Trigeminal	Sensory/general sensation from the face and anterior tongue; motor – muscles of mastication (masseter and temporalis)	Impaired mastication which can lead to difficulty forming bolus	Lightly touch points on client's face and tongue and ask if they can feel any pressure Ask client to open jaw against resistance Look for lack of symmetry with jaw movements
VII Facial	Taste from the anterior two thirds of tongue; innervates the salivary glands (except parotid); innervates muscles of the face (therefore important for facial expression); important for lip closure, innervates digastric muscle which is important for hyoid elevation	Impaired lip seal Reduced hyoid elevation Decreased amount of saliva	Taste testing Look for facial paralysis: wrinkle forehead, smile, kiss, whistle, puff out cheeks

| IX & X Glosso-pharyngeal and Vagus | Sensation from the posterior third of the tongue, the soft palate, palatine tonsils, pillars of fauces and pharynx; taste from the posterior third of the tongue; innervates the parotid gland; innervates most laryngeal and all pharyngeal muscles (except the stlylopharyngeous, which is innervated by the glossopharyngeal); innervates the greater part of the digestive tract and other abdominal viscera. Cardiac branches act to slow the rate of heartbeat; bronchial branch acts to constrict the bronchi; and its oesophageal branches control involuntary muscles in the oesophagus, stomach, gallbladder, pancreas, and small intestine, stimulating peristalsis and gastrointestinal secretions. Controls muscles for voice and the soft palate | Potential difficulty forming bolus Reduced pharyngeal motility Movement of base of tongue to pharyngeal wall reduced Silent aspiration Weak cough when aspiration occurs Impaired opening of upper oesophageal sphincter | Gag reflex is sometimes assessed; however, it is important to note that many people with no neurological history do not have a gag reflex Symmetry of soft palate elevation when saying 'aaah' – palate will deviate towards the unaffected side Voice quality – hoarseness Weak cough Endoscopy may indicate vocal cord paralysis |

| XII
Hypo-
glossal | Innervates muscles of the tongue (except for the palatoglossus, which is innervated by the vagus) | Difficulty forming bolus

Decreased movement of base of tongue to pharyngeal wall | Deviation of tongue to weak side

Deep furrowing indicating wastage of affected side of tongue

Weak tongue when pushed sideways against a spatula or into cheek against clinician's hand

Reduced agility when asked to move tongue side to side and repeat sounds, e.g. 'pa-ta-ka'

May sound 'dysarthric' |

Direct students to the following:

Cichero & Murdoch (2006) pages 12–21
Daniels & Huckabee (2008) pages 32–39 and 73–79
Groher & Crary (2010) pages 20–30
Logemann (1998) pages 322–323
Winstock (2005) pages 15–16

2. Write down how you would go about investigating cranial nerve function in (i) an infant; (ii) a child with complex physical and learning needs; and (iii) an adult with receptive aphasia.

(i) **An infant**: Before seeing the baby, look at the medical file. Important information to check includes APGAR scores, gestational age, birth weight and any significant medical issues. Observation of the baby is essential, including when the infant is at rest. Other situations to be observed such as deep sleep, active sleep, quiet alert, active awake, drowsy awake, and so on will provide additional information about general status. Parent reports of how the baby presents will also be essential. The baby's facial features need to be observed at rest. Then a non-nutritive examination needs to be carried out with examination of early infant reflexes such as: rooting reflex, biting reflex, gagging reflex, etc. Finally, an assessment of how the baby organizes sucking, breathing and swallowing needs to be undertaken.

(ii) **A child with complex physical and learning needs**: Before seeing the child, information on the child's eating and drinking history and learning development needs to be completed with the parents, carers and other relevant health, educational and social care practitioners. In addition, information about how the child communicates and their level of understanding needs to be gained as augmentative and alternative communication may be needed as part of the assessment and ongoing intervention plan. The child is likely to have a learning disability, so asking him/her to carry out commands such as 'Open your mouth' may be challenging. Therefore, observation at rest before eating needs to take place, with some manipulation, followed by close observation during a mealtime. Is the child able to feed themselves independently or do they require help? Are there any risk factors evident during the mealtime and, if so, what are they? Further assessment could explore how the child manages different textures and viscosities of food.

(iii) **An adult with receptive aphasia**: Before seeing the client, obtain as much information as you can about the client's level of understanding and what facilitates the client's understanding, e.g. writing key words, pictures, gestures. It is important that after introducing yourself you indicate why you are going to ask the client to do some movements. If they do not understand, support them with the relevant facilitation strategies, e.g. gesture, pictures, and written words. Ensure you use simple short instructions and use the facilitation strategies to help them to understand the instructions. If the facilitation strategies do not help, try demonstrating the required movement and asking them to copy.

Direct students to the following:

Winstock (2005), chapter 6, pages 55–58

3. Fill in the following table.

Oral phase disorders	**Clinical signs:** Drooling and spillage from lips Prolonged oral phase Difficulty forming bolus Multiple swallows Pooling and pocketing in oral cavities post swallow
	Observations you would expect when viewing VFSS/FEES: Difficulty forming bolus Reduced bolus propulsion Prolonged oral phase
	Possible causes: Reduced strength of lip seal Impaired tongue movement
Pharyngeal disorders	**Clinical signs:** Premature spillage over back of tongue Delayed swallow Multiple swallows Coughing Wet voice Reduced laryngeal elevation
	Observations you would expect when viewing VFSS/FEES: Reduced movement of base of tongue to pharyngeal wall Poorly coordinated swallow Asymmetry Pharyngeal residue and pooling
	Possible causes: Impaired movement of base of tongue Impaired pharyngeal movement Reduced laryngeal elevation

Aspiration	Clinical signs:
	Wet voice
	Cough
	Temperature spike
	Change in lung status
	Wheeze and crackles in lungs
	Low oxygen saturation levels
	Difficulties breathing
	Observations you would expect when viewing VFSS/FEES:
	Liquid penetrates to level below vocal cords

Direct students to the following:

Cichero & Murdoch (2006), page 512
Daniels & Huckabee (2008), chapter 15, pages 181–205
Groher & Crary (2010), pages 72–98 and 182–185
Logemann (1998), pages 73–76 and 167

4. Describe the difficulties associated with a weak base of tongue.

Premature spillage of liquid over the back of the tongue into the pharynx and incomplete bolus clearance due to limited ability of the tongue to help effective expulsion of the bolus into the pharyngeal phase. This could lead to an extended oral phase. There may also be residue remaining in the valleculae. Tongue base movement helps facilitate epiglottic closure.

Direct students to the following:

Cichero & Murdoch (2006), pages 206, 221 and 274
Groher & Crary (2010), pages 107–108
Logemann (1998), pages 79–80

5. What causes nasal regurgitation?

Impaired soft palate/velum function, reduced velo-pharyngeal closure.
May also, in some cases indicate difficulties further down the pharynx.

Direct students to the following:

Groher & Crary (2010), pages164
Logemann (1998), pages 96–97 and 323
Cichero & Murdoch (2006), pages 149, 246, 251 and 368

6. What is the function of the lips in swallowing?

• Prevents food and drink spilling out of the oral cavity.

• Is important for bolus formation in the oral stage of the swallow.

• Contributes to maintaining effective intra-oral pressure.

Direct students to the following:

Groher & Crary (2010), page 225
Logemann (1998), page 78
Winstock (2005), pages 8–9

7. What is the function of the epiglottis in swallowing?

Closes off and protects the airway during the pharyngeal stage of the swallow. It also directs food around the sides of airway.

Direct students to the following:

Groher & Crary (2010), pages 21–22
Cichero & Murdoch (2006), page 3
Logemann (1998), page 35

8. What happens if the upper oesophageal sphincter does not open during swallowing?

• Pooling of food or drink in piriform sinuses

• Increased risk of aspiration post-swallow

Direct students to the following:

Groher & Crary (2010), pages 26 and 29–30
Cichero & Murdoch (2006), page103, 202 and 203
Logemann (1998) page 35

9. This is a diagram of the adult anatomy. Write down three key features as to how this DIFFERS from an infant's anatomy.

- The infant larynx is sited high in the neck and is close to the soft palate and epiglottis

- The infant tongue appears to fill the oral cavity. It is in close approximation to the soft palate and cheeks

- The lower jaw of the infant is small and retracted in appearance

Direct students to the following:

Cichero & Murdoch (2006), pages 29–31
Groher & Crary (2010), pages 46–49
Winstock (2005), pages 12–16

10. Describe what you would expect (i) an infant; (ii) a 6-month-old child; (iii) a 12-month-old child; (iv) an 18-month-old child; and (v) a 24-month-old child to be eating?

(i) An infant will be receiving milk either from their mother's breast or from a bottle, or both.

(ii) A 6-month-old can take mashed foods and finger foods such as rusks under supervision. A more vertical tongue-tip pattern with less jaw movement is evident. The 6-month-old can bite food placed to the sides of the mouth. Sucking occurs once food gets onto tongue and mixes with saliva. Drinking skills from other utensils are beginning to develop and, initially, liquid loss is common as the jaw moves up and down and the tongue moves forward and backward. The tongue may protrude slightly on occasion. Self feeding, such as holding the bottle or lipped cup without help and finger feeding are developing.

(iii) A 12-month-old can cope with the introduction of chopped foods with an increasing variety of textures becoming evident. Children of this age can manage thicker textures as well as tolerate changes in utensils such as use of a flatter bowled spoon, for example. The tongue can transfer food from side to side of oral cavity. The gag is less sensitive and the upper lip is active in moving food from a spoon. In terms of oral motor skills and drinking, the tongue moves forward and backward. It may protrude beneath the cup to provide stability. Independent use of spoons and cups increase but the child may still require help from an adult to model and support the skill development.

(iv) At 18 months a child should be able to tolerate and chew firmer foods. A controlled bite should be developing. Chewing development would be ongoing with periodic episodes of lip closure when eating. Use of a cup is becoming established, with an up–down suck pattern with drinking. Jaw stability in relation to cup drinking is emerging at this time. A child may be able to get his cup to his mouth well, but his ability to tip the cup consistently and in a more refined way may not be evident. With the spoon, the child should be attempting to feed themselves and may well maintain getting the spoon into their mouth without turning it.

(iv) A 24-month-old child can chew firmer food and is able to use a controlled sustained bite on, e.g. biscuit, as well as chewing with lips closed at times. He may lose food or saliva when chewing. In terms of independence he gradually gets the spoon to his mouth without turning it, and he can lift his cup to his mouth but may tip too much, causing spillage. At some point during this stage, he will progress to using a cup without spilling as much fluid.

Direct students to the following:

Cichero & Murdoch (2006), pages 26–38
Groher & Crary (2010), pages 43–49
Winstock (2005), pages 4–24

11. Describe a minimum of four key features within an adult or a paediatric population that would predispose you to consider that the client had aspiration.

- Wet voice after drinking
- Cough after eating and/or drinking
- Temperature spike
- Change in lung status
- Persistent respiratory illness
- Eyes filling with tears during eating and/or drinking
- Facial colour change when eating and/or drinking
- Wheeze and crackles in lungs
- Low oxygen saturation levels
- Difficulties breathing
- Delayed swallow reflex
- Drowsiness
- Excess oral residue

Direct students to the following:

Cichero & Murdoch (2006), pages 415 and 512
Groher & Crary (2010), pages 5–6 and 182–185
Logemann (1998), page 167
Winstock (2005), page 31

12. Describe a non-instrumental dysphagia assessment that can be used for an adult or a child. Describe the key features that are observed and evaluated when using this assessment. It may be helpful to consider a commercially available assessment, for example, the MASA: Mann Assessment of Swallowing by Giselle Mann (2002), or the SOMA: Schedule of Oral Motor Assessment by Sheena Reilly et al. (2000).

Informal assessment can include:

Target	Elicitation	Observations
Facial symmetry	Have subject look straight at you	Are all facial features symmetrical?
Lips	Smile Pucker Open Close tight Puff up cheeks, hold against resistance	Look for symmetrical movements, extent of movements, ability to close lips completely, and hold against resistance
Tongue	Stick straight out Left Right Left and right quickly Elevation Protrusion and lateral movement against resistance (with tongue blade) Didokinetic rate	Look for symmetry and range of motion. Look at size of tongue and for evidence of unusual movements. Assess ability to exert force against resistance. Assess coordination of fast movements
Oral cavity	Open wide	Look at teeth, tongue, hard and soft palate. Look for evidence of lesions, atrophy, or missing structures Look for signs of poor oral care Also observe jaw excursion, listen for 'clicks', watch for unusual movements

Velum	Say 'ah'	Watch for extent and symmetry of velar elevation and pharyngeal constriction
Voice	Maximum phonation time Pitch glides	Listen for vocal intensity, pitch, quality and signs of reduced breath support
Pharynx	Feel the larynx at rest and when saliva is swallowed Feel the larynx again when the client is drinking water, and when eating semi-solids	Feel for any indication of impaired timing of movement, uncoordination or reduced movement Listen and look for any signs of aspiration before, during and after a swallow

Reference to cranial nerve function in relation to informal oral motor assessment can include further information on differentiation between upper and lower motor neurone difficulties:

CN V: Lower motor neurone difficulties would include a weakness and deviation to one side, and muscle atrophy.

Upper motor neurone difficulties would include a more mild and possibly a transitory weakness.

CN VII: Lower motor neurone difficulties would include a one-sided facial weakness, a limited range of movement of the articulators and taste/sensation difficulties.

Upper motor neurone difficulties would include limited lip and neck muscle movement, difficulties with forehead wrinkling, and decreased taste sensation.

CN IX: Lower motor neurone difficulties would include no gag on stimulation in the oral cavity (however, it is important to note that absence of a gag reflex is not an accurate measure as many healthy people have an absent gag reflex), limited or restricted palatal function, an absent or delayed swallow and poor voice quality.

Upper motor neurone difficulties would include limited palatal movement and pharyngeal control, a harsh voice quality, delayed or absent swallow and aspiration/penetration.

CN X: Lower motor neurone difficulties would include flaccid muscle tone as the nerve fibres travelling from the anterior horn of the spinal cord to the muscles have been affected.

Upper motor neurone difficulties would include a spastic muscle tone as the lesion would be *above* the anterior horn cell or motor nuclei of the cranial nerves.

CN XII: Lower motor neurone difficulties would include atrophy, fasciculation, weakness, deviation of tongue to side of lesion and decreased tone.

Upper motor neurone difficulties would include weakness, reduced range of movement of the articulators, increased tone, imprecise movements and deviation of tongue to contra-lateral side.

1. Mann, G. (2002) *MASA: The Mann Assessment of Swallowing Ability.* New York: Thompson Delmar Learning.

This assessment is designed for use in bedside evaluations of patients referred for swallowing function assessment. It is appropriate for a range of adult clients. This tool may also be utilized for monitoring swallowing skills over time. Patients are assessed on the following: alertness, cooperation, comprehension, respiration, respiratory rate for swallow, dysphasia, dyspraxia, dysarthria, saliva, lip seal, tongue movement, tongue strength, tongue coordination, oral preparation, gag, palate, bolus clearance, oral transit time, cough reflex, voluntary cough, voice, tracheostomy tube present and type, pharyngeal phase, pharyngeal response and likelihood of aspiration.

2. Reilly, S., Skuse, D., & Wolke. D. (2000) *Schedule for Oral Motor Assessment – SOMA.* Whurr Publishers, London & Philadelphia.

The SOMA has four main components: (i) oral motor challenge categories; (ii) functional areas being investigated; (iii) functional units/activity of the muscle groups; and (iv) discrete oral motor behaviour.

Direct students to the following:

Cichero & Murdoch (2006), pages 147–190
Daniels & Huckabee (2008), pages 53–108

Logemann (1998), pages 135–186
Winstock (2005), pages 104–127
Mann (2002), *MASA: The Mann Assessment of Swallowing Ability*. Thompson Delmar Learning, New York
Reilly, S., Skuse, D., & Wolke. D. (2000), *Schedule for Oral Motor Assessment – SOMA*. Whurr Publishers, London & Philadelphia

13. What is a videofluoroscopic swallowing study, and what are the criteria for using this instrumental evaluation as an assessment tool?

A videofluoroscopic swallowing study (VFSS) is a radiological procedure and provides a video x-ray of a client's swallowing status. Barium is used so that food and liquid can be identified as clearly as possible on the video x-ray. During this procedure, the speech and language therapist will often trial different strategies, and different consistencies and textures. Compared with a bedside assessment, this procedure can usually more objectively investigate whether aspiration has occurred and can usually allow a more objective evaluation of the oral and pharyngeal phases of the swallow. It can also be used to ascertain the most appropriate texture and fluid modification to be used with a client, and can also be used to develop strategies for compensation.

Criteria for using: When appropriate diagnosis and management decisions cannot be made from non-instrumental assessment alone, e.g. the clinician may suspect silent aspiration or may need further information about the anatomy and physiology of the swallow before recommending a particular management approach.

Direct students to the following:

Cichero & Murdoch (2006), pages 191–212
Daniels & Huckabee (2008), pages 119–140
Groher & Crary (2010), pages 195–199 and 201
Logemann (1998), pages 58–61, 168–189 and 360
Winstock (2005), pages 122–125

14. Compare the following assessments: videofluoroscopic swallowing study and fibreoptic endoscopic evaluation of swallowing. What are two key advantages and disadvantages of each of these approaches?

VFSS

Advantages: Good lateral view of the phases of the swallow; duration of the phases assessed; viscosity safety can be assessed in relation to fluids and textures; images can be kept and reviewed later.

Limitations: Radiation risk; barium alters true viscosity and taste of everyday foods; artificial setting, not a real mealtime context; local problems with access to VFSS; seating; not pleasant for children; not appropriate for obese clients; not appropriate for agitated or confused clients; only snapshot in time; not appropriate for clients who have difficulties travelling; process of getting to VFSS suite may result in fatigue which may impact on swallow; may not capture impact of fatigue on swallow as does not assess an entire mealtime.

FEES

Advantages: Portable; no radiation; can use everyday foods without adding anything to it (although some therapists add food dye so liquids and food can be more clearly seen); can see larynx and see clearly issues with secretions; can use in a therapy session.

Limitations: Invasive; requires additional training; unable to see critical phase of the swallow, so you will be using your own clinical judgement (this is because the view of the larynx is obscured by the pharyngeal walls and epiglottic inversion during the swallow); aspiration is *assumed* from coating rather than seeing the aspiration; hard to gain information re the oesophageal phase, although inferences can be made. Not appropriate for agitated clients.

Direct students to the following:

Cichero & Murdoch (2006), pages 191–234
Daniels & Huckabee (2008), pages 119–140 and 158
Groher & Crary (2010), pages 195–199, 201–205 and 281–282

Logemann (1998), pages 54–61 and 168–189
Winstock (2005), page 121

15. Describe three management and/or therapy approaches that you have read about for an adult dysphagia caseload, or three management and/or therapy approaches for a paediatric caseload.

Students should consider the following:

Adult caseload

- Postural changes
- Manoeuvres
- Thermal and tactile stimulation
- Dietary modifications
- Fluid modifications
- Alternate sources of feeding, e.g. PEG
- Medications, e.g. saliva management, anti-reflux
- Surgical
- Botox
- Oral hygiene
- Equipment
- Training of others

Paediatric caseload

- Non-nutritive sucking
- Positioning
- Desensitization programmes
- Increasing sensory awareness programmes
- Texture modification programmes for both fluids and solids

- Pacing
- Oral control support programmes
- Intra-oral appliances
- Chewing programmes
- Equipment presentation, e.g. lateral spoon presentation, dummy spoon presentation (to clear a bolus)
- Messy play programmes
- Training of others

Direct students to the following:

Cichero & Murdoch (2006), pages 319–342, 466 and 487–540
Daniels & Huckabee (2008), pages 207–305
Groher & Crary (2010), pages 231–307
Logemann (1998), pages191–250, 275–276, 297 and 345–357
Winstock (2005), pages 128–162

16. Some medications can have an impact on appetite and/or swallowing. Typically, such medications include anti-convulsants, analgesics, anti-depressants and tranquillisers. Carry out a search to investigate how medication can impact on a specific client group and write down your findings. Consider the side effects and the potential effect on the swallow. An example could be the anti-convulsant Phenytoin. This can cause nausea and vomiting, but can also contribute to poor oral motor control and uncoordinated swallowing.

Examples include:

CNS depressants, e.g. barbiturates – delayed swallow, impaired coordination at oral stage, sedation

Anti-convulsants, e.g. Phenytoin, ethosuximide – delayed swallow, impaired coordination at oral and pharyngeal stage

Anti-Parkinsonian, e.g. Levodopa – difficulties with bolus control, impaired pharyngeal motility, cricopharyngeal dysfunction, impaired pharyngeal stage

Narcotic analgesics, e.g. morphine – delayed swallow, impaired coordination at oral stage, sedation

Direct students to the following:

Cichero & Murdoch (2006), pages 249, 252, 254 and 289–298
Groher & Crary (2010), pages 15, 138, 156–158 and 239
Logemann (1998), pages 312–313 and 368–370
Winstock (2005), page 42

Pre-placement Quiz 2:
Oral hygiene and aspiration pneumonia

1. Why is oral hygiene an important consideration in the management of infants, children and adults with dysphagia?

Poor oral hygiene is a risk factor for pneumonia. This risk is increased when the client has dysphagia as the pathogens found in the mouths of clients with poor oral hygiene can be aspirated.

2. What are some of the risk factors for aspiration pneumonia?

Reliance on others for feeding

Tube feeding

Dysphagia

Poor oral hygiene

Dependence on others for oral hygiene

More than one medical diagnosis

Taking many medications

Smoking

3. What do a healthy mouth and healthy gums look like?

Gums are pale pink

Gums have clearly defined, shaped edges

Gums do not bleed easily

4.Why are people who have disabilities, dementia and/or are nil by mouth at high risk of having poor oral hygiene?

They are reliant on others to provide oral hygiene. Carers often do not have adequate training and are often rushed so do not provide appropriate care. Clients may have behavioural issues and this may mean that the process of cleaning their mouth may be very difficult for carers. Clients with poor cognition may find it difficult to understand the importance of oral hygiene. Clients with dysphagia have an increased risk of being dehydrated which is a significant risk factor for poor oral hygiene.

Difficulties associated with determining most appropriate method, e.g. clients with dysphagia may aspirate mouth wash. Clients with dysphagia also may have reduced frequency of saliva clearance which may result in a build-up of bacteria. Some medications can also impact on saliva production and clearance which can also lead to a build-up of bacteria. Tube feeding is often associated with poor oral hygiene.

5. What should you do if you notice someone has poor oral hygiene?

Inform your supervisor or clinical educator. Inform the relevant multidisciplinary team and alert them to the risks associated with poor oral hygiene. If appropriate, refer to dentistry.

6. What are some of the challenges associated with maintaining good oral hygiene in people who have dysphagia and communication disabilities?

They may have difficulties in understanding why oral hygiene is important. It is often difficult for health professionals to adequately communicate appropriate strategies.

7. What are some strategies for overcoming these challenges?

Work with the MDT in order to facilitate understanding. Produce materials that are more accessible for people with communication difficulties.

Direct students to:

http://www.cetl.org.uk/learning/OHI_dysphagia/player.html

About the contributors

Naomi Cocks is a Senior Lecturer, Clinical Tutor and Clinical Educator in the Department of Language and Communication Science at City University London. She lectures on dysphagia to pre-registration students and qualified speech and language therapists. Naomi trained at Curtin University of Technology in Perth, Australia. Prior to becoming a lecturer, Naomi worked in Australia as a speech pathologist in a range of settings including acute, rehabilitation and community facilities. In these settings, she assessed and managed adult clients with a range of swallowing difficulties and also supervised many students.

Celia Harding is a Senior Lecturer and Clinical Tutor in the Department of Language and Communication Science, City University London. She is also a speech and language therapist and continues to practise at the Royal Free Hospital as part of the paediatric gastroenterology team. She teaches in the areas of learning disability and paediatric dysphagia both at pre- and post-registration level.

Annie Aloysius is a Senior Clinical Specialist Speech and Language Therapist at Imperial College Healthcare NHS Trust, London. She works on the neonatal units at Queen Charlottes and St Mary's Hospitals and has significant experience working with paediatric dysphagia, specializing in preterm feeding and recently adding the qualification of Lactation Consultant to her clinical skills. Previously, she worked with children with congenital neuromuscular disease. She teaches regularly and has a number of publications in her areas of clinical interest.

Lesley Baker qualified as a speech and language therapist in 2000 from Queen Margaret University College, Edinburgh. After working for four years in paediatric community clinics and special schools in West Hertfordshire, she moved to the Bobath Centre for Children with Cerebral Palsy where she worked until 2008. She is trained in the Bobath approach. In 2008, she started working for the Complex Motor Disorders Service at the Evelina Children's Hospital where her remit is assessing children and young people with complex motor disorders for the suitability of specialized neurosurgical interventions of deep brain stimulation (DBS) for dystonia or an intrathecal baclofen (ITB) pump implantation for mixed spasticity and dystonia, as well as following these children up post-surgery. She also treats some acute paediatric inpatients and jointly runs the trust's paediatric videofluoroscopic swallow study clinic. She is a London Paediatric Dysphagia Special Interest Group committee member.

Nina Bharania qualified as a speech and language therapist in 2004 from the University of Central England in Birmingham. She has previous experience of working with children and young people in special schools and now works full time with Adults with Learning Disabilities (ALD) as Dysphagia Lead for Barnet Learning Disabilities Service in North London. In 2010, she qualified in Advanced Clinical Practice in Dysphagia, specializing in ALD. With a special interest in training, Nina has developed and coordinated in-house dysphagia training for speech and language therapists across all adult community settings in Barnet and has recently joined the team of tutors on the Adults with Learning Disabilities Special Interest Group Dysphagia Course. Nina maintains a varied clinical caseload as well as coordinating and developing the dysphagia service in Barnet and supervising junior staff and students.

Helen Cockerill is a Consultant Speech and Language Therapist in the Paediatric Neurosciences Department at the Evelina Children's Hospital (part of Guy's and St Thomas' NHS Foundation Trust). She has over 27 years of experience of feeding children with cerebral palsy and other motor disabilities, and in managing complex communication disorders, including the use of Augmentative and Alternative Communication. She has also developed an interest in behavioural feeding difficulties associated with autism, learning disability and complex medical conditions. She teaches and writes, in an attempt to share her experience before she forgets it all.

Stacey Lawrence is a speech and language therapist who has a broad experience in working with infants and children with a range of eating and drinking difficulties. She jointly developed a dysphagia competency and training protocol for SLTs in her capacity as Dysphagia lead for schools in a large community team in Harrow. She currently works in the field of acute paediatric and neonatal feeding across Imperial College Healthcare NHS Trust. This work also includes supporting a well-established multidisciplinary feeding clinic.

Michelle Miles qualified as a speech and language therapist from University College London in 2001. After working for several years in community paediatric dysphagia and communication in Enfield and Waltham Forest, she moved to the acute setting at the Evelina Children's Hospital in 2009.

Michelle works as part of a team of inpatient speech and language therapists and her clinical remit is to take a lead role in the neurology and cardiology specialities, assessing and managing infants and children with dysphagia and complex communication difficulties.

Lizzie Nash qualified as a speech and language therapist from University College London in 1999. Since then, she has worked as a speech and language therapist in the NHS. Her early experience was in Bristol, working with children with developmental feeding and communication difficulties in a range of community settings, including special schools and language units. Lizzie worked at Great Ormond Street Children's Hospital for five years in the multidisciplinary team that supported the needs of children with tracheostomies. She combined this with a position as Clinical and Professional Skills Module Coordinator/Clinical Tutor on the MSc course at University College London. Following a stint working with a broader paediatric and neonatal caseload at St George's Hospital, Lizzie moved to her current full-time post at Evelina Children's Hospital where she leads the acute team of speech and language therapists. Her clinical remit is to develop the speech and language therapy service to neonates, infants and children with complex airway conditions. Lizzie completed an MSc in 2008; her research investigated the characteristics of supraglottic voice, a way of achieving phonation observed in a group of children following laryngotracheal reconstruction surgery.

Camille Paynter graduated with honours as a speech pathologist from La Trobe University Melbourne in 2001, and worked in adult neurological rehabilitation in the private health sector before moving to the UK in 2006. At the Whittington Hospital, London, she was Clinical Lead (Adult Service) for four years where she worked with patients with acquired swallowing and communication disorders, supervised a team of speech and language therapists, and coordinated the student placement programme. Camille also developed her interest in clinical ethics sitting on the hospital's Clinical Ethics Group. She has a strong interest in student clinical education and supervises students both on clinical placements and as a Visiting Clinical Tutor for City University London. Camille is presently a speech and language therapist at the National Hospital for Neurology and Neurosurgery, London, working with adult patients with acquired and progressive neurological conditions.